DK Na

Sec

QIGONG

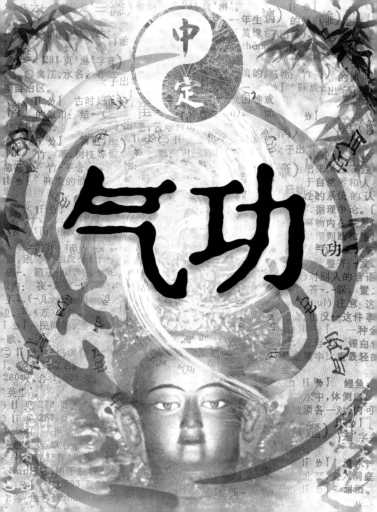

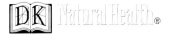

Secrets of

QIGONG

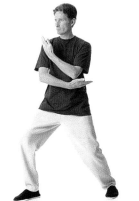

CONSULTANT

ANGUS CLARK

DK Publishing, Inc.

DK

LONDON, NEW YORK, SYDNEY, DELHI, PARIS, MUNICH, and JOHANNESBURG

First published in The United States of America in 2001 by
DK PUBLISHING, INC.,
95 Madison Avenue, New York, New York 10016

Text by Helen Varley

Art director *Peter Bridgewater*
Publisher *Sophie Collins*
Editorial director *Steve Luck*
Designers *Kevin Knight, Alistair Plumb*
Picture researcher *Vanessa Fletcher*
Photography *Guy Ryecart*
Illustrations *Coral Mula, Ivan Hissey, Rhian Nest-James,*
Michael Courtney, Sandy Gardner

This book was conceived, designed, and produced by
THE IVY PRESS LIMITED,
The Old Candlemakers, Lewes,
East Sussex, England, BN7 2NZ

Natural Health ® is a registered trademark of Weider
Publications, Inc. *Natural Health Magazine* is the leading
publication in the field of natural self-care. For subscription
information call 800–526–8440 or visit
www.naturalhealthmag.com

Copyright © 2001 The Ivy Press Limited

All rights reserved under International and Pan-American
Copyright Conventions. No part of this publication may be
reproduced, stored in a retrieval system, or transmitted in
any form or by any means, electronic, mechanical,
photocopying, recording, or otherwise, without the prior
written permission of the copyright owner. Published in
Great Britain by DK Limited.

A Cataloging in Publication record is
available from the Library of Congress
ISBN 0-7894-7782-3

Originated and printed by
Hong Kong Graphics and
Printing Limited, China

see our complete
catalog at

www.dk.com

CONTENTS

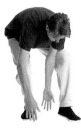

Flowing movements
The sequence of movements in Chapter 4 is divided into separate, self-contained exercises for ease of learning.

HOW TO USE THIS BOOK

The *Secrets of QiGong* is a startup guide for newcomers to QiGong, and a useful handbook for teachers and more experienced students to use for practice between classes. It explains the basics of learning QiGong—energy flow, posture and alignment, movement, and the role of the mind—and it presents a sequence of 128 classic QiGong movements or exercises. Its five chapters also give a useful introduction to an ancient Eastern art that has proved its relevance to 21st-century living.

At a Glance

Chapter 1 explores the ancient Chinese origins of QiGong

Chapter 2 looks at life energy or Qi—the foundation of QiGong

Chapter 3 explains what you need and prepares you for QiGong practice

Chapter 4 presents a classic QiGong movement sequence to exercise body and mind, promote health, and prevent illness and disease.

Chapter 5 explains how you can use QiGong in daily life.

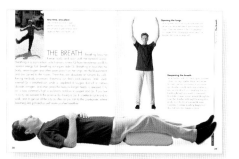

The basics
The first chapters look at life energy and its pathways through the body, breathing, stance, and movement.

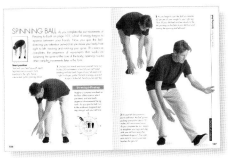

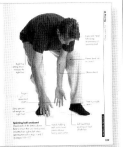

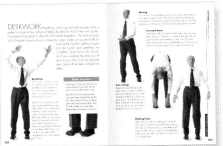

How to Use this Book

The exercises

Full-color pages show each exercise in detail, with an introduction explaining the purpose and health-giving benefits of each movement. Numbered captions explain how to perform each step in sequence, and details are shown in closeup.

Analysis

Black-and-white pages analyze each exercise. The text describes the movement sequence, annotated images pinpoint the positioning of each body part, and drawings illustrate the role of the mind's eye in the exercise.

The wider world

Chapter 5 shows you how to make Qigong relevant to your daily life with a series of short exercise programs to increase your energy at work, to deal with the demands of others, and to defuse aggression in yourself and from others.

Introduction

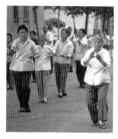

QiGong in China

Like taiji (t'ai chi), QiGong is a Chinese system of exercises to promote health and longevity. Chinese people often practice QiGong in groups out in the open.

QiGong exercises and movements are designed to conserve and build energy. The practice of QiGong originated in China, where it evolved over thousands of years. Eventually, during the 20th century, knowledge of the art reached the West, and it is now spreading rapidly across the world.

Practicing QiGong stimulates the body's energy levels through postural exercises and slow, gentle movements that activate the circulation of blood along arteries and veins, and the flow of life energy or Qi along its channels or meridians. It exercises but does not tire joints, tendons, and muscles. QiGong also involves learning to use the mind to guide Qi to parts of the body where it is needed to strengthen and heal.

A healing art

This invigorating form of exercise may be practiced from the teen years up to the last day of your life. The movements are slow and do not stress or strain the body, so you can begin at any age. And you gain immediate benefits, however unfit you are when you begin. Lifelong practice ensures mobility into old age. In fact, QiGong is said to have the power to extend life. The form or sequence of exercises presented in Chapter 4 is based on the movements of the White Crane, the ancient Chinese symbol of longevity.

It is possible to begin learning QiGong alone by following the instructions in this book, but at some stage you will need to find a teacher who will show you how to practice most effectively, and help you move on. People who are bedridden or who use crutches or wheelchairs can benefit from QiGong, but they need a teacher's guidance on practicing safely. Pregnant women need to follow gentle exercises supervised by a qualified teacher.

QiGong can be a useful tool for day-to-day living, improving concentration and restoring some of the feeling and spontaneity we had as children. It has many forms and branches, some of which can lead to self-exploration and meditation. Whatever you hope to get from it, expect QiGong to introduce something special into your life.

Safety

Always consult a physician before beginning any program of exercise, especially if you have a long-standing medical condition, if you are undergoing treatment, or if you have recently had surgery, an injury, or medical treatment. Pregnant women should not practice the form exercises in Chapter 4. QiGong can be used to treat many illnesses and medical conditions, but only under the supervision of a qualified and experienced QiGong teacher.

ROOTS

QiGong is rapidly becoming known in the West as an effective system of exercise for combating stress, preventing disease, and promoting fitness and relaxation. In China, where it originated and evolved, it is widely practiced for health and longevity. Chapter 1 tells the story of QiGong, exploring its ancient origins. Many of its techniques were preserved for generations as clan or family secrets until the 20th century when the veil of secrecy was lifted and masters of the art offered their knowledge to a wider audience. By the close of the century it had spread to the West, where it is now widely practiced.

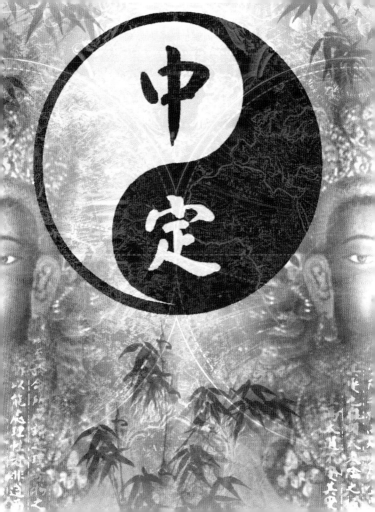

What Is QiGong?

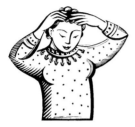

Anmogong

QiGong involves many different healing actions. Self-massage, a technique called anmogong, has an important healing role.

QiGong (or chi gung or chi kung) means "energy work" and essentially, it is the art of cultivating Qi to promote health and vitality. Qi is the energy of life, the energy, once called "ether," which has inhabited the universe since time began and which pervades everything in it. Qi is the energy that drives the planets along their orbits, and it fills the Earth, and the air, the rocks, and the rivers.

Qi is the vital force in all living things, the life force in the human body and mind. QiGong is an approach to exercise that works to build and maintain the body's store of Qi and ensure its free circulation everywhere in the body. Many factors impede the flow of Qi, from ignorance and depression to inactivity, fatigue, poor diet, stress, and pollution. QiGong seeks to reeducate mind and body through exercise and self-exploration, encouraging new ways of living that will counter their effects.

There are many different styles of QiGong, all having evolved different movements, but each one begins with a range of core exercises that fall into two types. The first consists of exercises in which you do not move your body visibly. These are quiescent or static exercises and they work on posture, realigning parts of the body to facilitate the flow of Qi. All QiGong exercises have a strong mental component, and quiescent exercises often involve a meditation. The dynamic exercises, the second category, are movements. They are designed to mobilize joints, stretch tendons, strengthen muscles, and improve balance and coordination. But QiGong movements are slow, even, steady, and graceful, demanding great muscle control without strain or impact. Dynamic exercises improve the circulation of blood and lymph, as well as of Qi. They release Qi stored in the body, expel used and stale Qi, and tap into energy circulating in the external world, in the Earth and the sky, to replenish the body's stores.

Linking body and mind

Visualizations always accompany moving postures. The mind learns to follow the flow of Qi along a meridian to or from an energy gateway—the point where it enters or leaves the body. The standing meditations are exercises in developing awareness of the role of Qi in and around the body. They teach you to control its flow and to direct the healing and vitalizing Qi energy to wherever it is needed in the body. This is the main aim of QiGong exercises.

ORIGINS OF QIGONG

QiGong may have originated in prehistoric times, for its birth is hidden in China's legendary ancient history. It may have developed hand in hand with the earliest healing systems; exercises for health appear in the classic writings attributed to the Yellow Emperor, considered the founder of Chinese medicine. Some historians attribute the origins of QiGong to dances of ancient peoples who believed rhythmic movement could remove stagnation and obstruction in the body. But some of the most important principles of QiGong were formulated by the Daoists, whose ideas emerged some 2,500 years ago and evolved into one of the principal schools of Chinese thought. They searched for an elixir of life and devised exercises to encourage the body's organs to manufacture one.

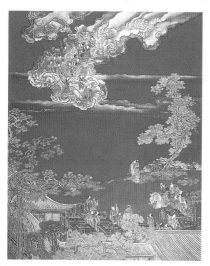

The Daoist Immortals
QiGong techniques developed by Daoists during the first millennium BC may have helped them resist illness and extend their lifespan beyond what was normal for the times, earning them their reputation as immortal beings with supernatural powers.

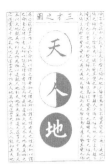

Life energy

The relationship between bodily energy and the energy of the cosmos and the Earth is shown in this ancient scroll.

Daoist thought

The legendary Daoist sage, Lao Tzu, shown right, is said to have written the Dao De Jing (Tao Te Ching), an anthology of writings by Daoist philosophers. They believed in valuing and preserving life and avoiding injury to the human body. Longevity was their ideal.

Martial Tradition

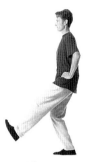

Martial movements
The kick on page 186 is a familiar movement in gong fu and in taijiquan fighting arts. In QiGong it is a way of releasing energy.

Q iGong is essentially a peaceful art, wholly concerned with health and healing. But it is thought to have evolved toward the end of the first millennium BC, a time of prolonged unrest in China when the Chinese martial arts may also have developed. Their origins, like those of QiGong, are lost in legend, but the first written references, from the AD 600s, refer to patterns of movement perhaps similar to QiGong movements. QiGong

could have helped fighters build and focus energy, increase their strength and stamina, and improve their coordination.

Daoist roots

Taijiquan (t'ai chi ch'uan) grew from the same Daoist roots as QiGong. Most Westerners know it as an exercise system aimed at ensuring good health and longevity. Posture, breathing, movement, and visualization are all part of it. But taijiquan evolved as a martial art: its movements may be adapted for fighting; it emphasizes practice with a partner, and it has weapons forms using staff and sword. It is called a soft or internal martial art because rather than use force against force, it focuses on gathering and directing energy, guided by the mind. According to legend, an early taiji teacher, Chang San-feng, studied among Daoists on the sacred Wudang Mountain, where he was inspired by the martial potential of yielding when he watched a snake fight a bird. Today, QiGong is commonly used in martial arts to cultivate energy.

The Shaolin tradition

Some historians claim that gong fu (kung fu) predates taijiquan, but the two martial styles may have common origins. Gong fu is a "hard" martial art—it relies on external strength and the use of force, as in punching and kicking, but QiGong techniques are used to strengthen joints and muscles and to achieve speed.

All gong fu styles are said to derive from fighting arts once taught in the ancient kingdom of Wei at the Shaolin Temple. During the AD mid-500s, an Indian Buddhist monk, Boddhidharma,

is said to have introduced to the fighting monks the new quiescent techniques of deep breathing and meditation. These they used to build mental strength in combat.

During the AD 600s Shaolin Temple boxing spread through China, influencing the development of the martial arts. Modern gong fu uses entirely different breathing techniques from taijiquan, but the historic influence of QiGong is evident in gong fu training to maximize a fighter's internal power.

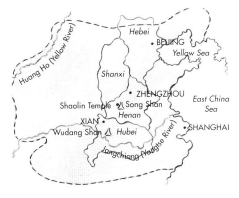

Cradle of Daoism

QiGong evolved rapidly during the first millennium BC, when China was a cluster of small, warring states extending across modern Hebei, Shanxi, Henan, and Hubei provinces. The Wudang Mountains became a retreat for Daoist recluses who developed the philosophical ideas on which QiGong is based.

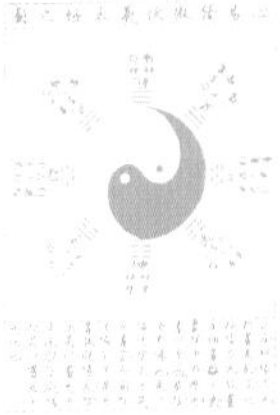

Taiji QiGong
This ancient diagram shows the close relationship between QiGong and taiji (t'ai chi). In the West they are now merging into a style, taiji QiGong.

QIGONG PATHWAYS
QiGong reached the West so recently that we talk as if there were only one form of QiGong. Yet the practice began as diverse techniques for managing Qi. Ancient writings describe more than 200, ranging from tuna, or the art of expelling and admitting Qi, to those with special healing potential, such as fang song gong relaxation, techniques to aid recovery from illness. Many different styles of QiGong evolved, from martial forms such as neigong—originally a way of training the mind to make the body more resistant to blows—to Daoist QiGong, a system for self-exploration and development.

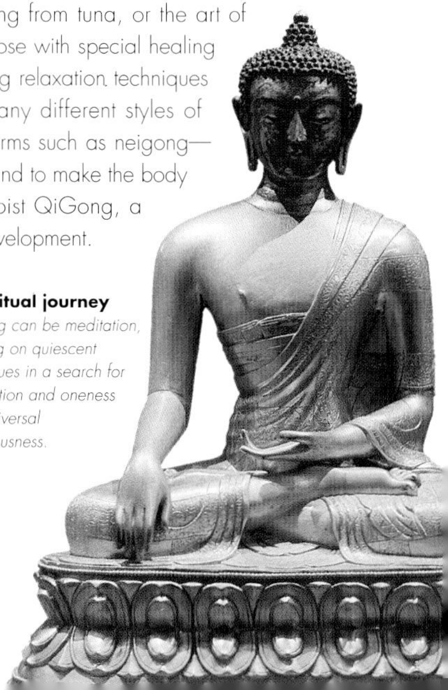

A spiritual journey
QiGong can be meditation, focusing on quiescent techniques in a search for purification and oneness with universal consciousness.

Buddhist QiGong

Buddhism spread widely in China after its introduction during the first millennium BC, and many Buddhist temples were built. A Buddhist school of QiGong subsequently developed in China.

Confucian QiGong

Followers of Confucian QiGong seek to develop moral virtues and to cultivate wisdom.

Global QiGong

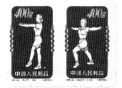

After the Revolution

Many styles of QiGong and taiji traditionally taught to a select few were made available for ordinary Chinese people to learn after 1949.

QiGong has been developing and evolving for some thousands of year. Many of its ancient techniques have been lost as a result of the destruction of temples and libraries, of cults and religions brought about during successive political upheavals in China. Much has been preserved, however, rediscovered in archeological sites, translated from ancient manuscripts, or simply passed on as folk knowledge. For centuries exercises for treating illness have been passed down orally from generation to generation of physicians who combined QiGong exercises with other traditional medical practices, often writing them as prescriptions in medical documents. Until recently, however, a large body of QiGong exercises was unavailable to most ordinary Chinese people. These were developed by families or clans with a martial tradition, who kept them, as part of their fighting techniques, as closely guarded secrets. In 1900, however, British troops first used firearms to devastating effect to put down the Boxer Rebellion in China, and men wielding guns rapidly replaced clans of men trained in the ancient fighting arts as defenders of villages or supporters of warring lords. Gradually, members of fighting clans relinquished their secrets and began to teach their fighting skills and pass on their QiGong techniques to outsiders.

QiGong travels West

Until the 1950s QiGong remained an exclusively Chinese art. It may have been known and practiced in the Chinese communities in Hong Kong, Malaysia, and other Asian countries, but was scarcely heard of in the West. After the Chinese Communist Revolution in 1949, a revival of ancient Chinese healing arts such as acupuncture, taijiquan, and QiGong was encouraged by the government under Chairman Mao Zedong. By the 1960s they had become commonly practiced among Chinese people and new, easy-to-learn forms, such as the now well-known QiGong form called Taiji Eighteen Steps, spread beyond the borders of China and even outside Asia to the West. During the 1970s, Westerners such as the American writer and teacher Bruce Frantzis studied in China under Chinese masters. He returned to the US to write and teach, disseminating his knowledge of QiGong to Westerners.

Bridge to the West
Dr. Chi Chiang-tao left China in the 1950s and taught taiji and QiGong to Western students until his death in 1995.

THE ART OF QI

QiGong is the art of using and controlling life energy, or Qi. According to ancient Chinese principles of healing, physical and mental fitness become possible only when sufficient Qi of the right quality is able to flow freely around the body along its designated pathways. ᥬ The objective of all QiGong exercises is to develop energy by facilitating the flow of Qi around the body. This chapter explains the ideas behind the practice of QiGong, from the ancient Chinese concepts of yin and yang, to Qi's effect on body functions, and the role of the mind, awareness, and visualization in exercise. QiGong is a holistic, healing art, a form of preventive medicine.

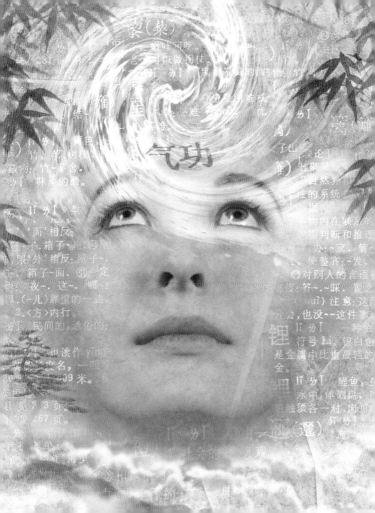

A Healing Practice

Most people say they start QiGong to maintain health and fitness, having heard that it keeps people healthy into old age. And some take it up with the aim of deepening their self-knowledge and maximizing their potential. QiGong is certainly therapeutic. If practiced regularly, its gentle movements exercise the joints without stressing or damaging them as high-impact sports can do, and this keeps degenerative diseases at bay. It is effective in restoring normal functioning to injured limbs and joints.

Medical benefits

Research carried out in the late 20th century indicates that QiGong may help reduce blood pressure, it may have a strengthening effect on the immune system, it may affect body chemistry beneficially through the endocrine system, and, in time, it appears to improve heart function. For many hundreds of years, masters of QiGong have, in addition, claimed that practicing QiGong can cure many serious diseases and disorders, and can extend the human life span well past its average length. Considerable research is needed before these claims can be proved to the satisfaction of Western physicians. Undoubtedly, however, the combination of deep breathing, concentration, and gentle exercise has a beneficial effect on many illnesses, and prevents the development of a range of stress-related diseases.

Effects on the mind

QiGong is a holistic system involving mind and body. Many people believe that it can improve mental ability and even cure mental illness. Certainly, depression, anxiety, and other emotional problems can be alleviated by concentration techniques and relaxation. QiGong is not a panacea, but in the destabilizing environment of 21st-century life it provides badly needed physical and emotional stability. All physicians, Western as well as Eastern, have long stressed the positive role of the mind in healing.

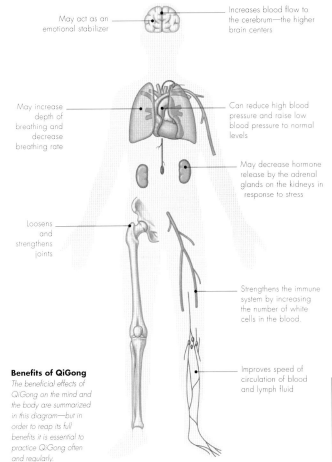

May act as an emotional stabilizer

Increases blood flow to the cerebrum—the higher brain centers

May increase depth of breathing and decrease breathing rate

Can reduce high blood pressure and raise low blood pressure to normal levels

May decrease hormone release by the adrenal glands on the kidneys in response to stress

Loosens and strengthens joints

Strengthens the immune system by increasing the number of white cells in the blood.

Improves speed of circulation of blood and lymph fluid

Benefits of QiGong

The beneficial effects of QiGong on the mind and the body are summarized in this diagram—but in order to reap its full benefits it is essential to practice QiGong often and regularly.

LIFE ENERGY

The Chinese word for energy is "Qi" ("chi"). Qi is the vital force that existed before the universe or living beings existed, whose movements gave rise to the stars and planets, to the Earth, nature, the weather, the oceans, and the land. Qi is the life force that inhabits all living things, fueling their growth, change, movements, actions, and thought. There are many different forms of Qi. There is the heavenly Qi from the sun and moon, and Qi from the Earth. There is the Qi humans are born with, and a healing Qi which QiGong masters can emit. Newcomers to QiGong may find it simpler to think in terms of external Qi, which inhabits the outside world, filling the sky and the Earth; and internal Qi, which circulates inside the human body, the force that gives it vitality, the energy that powers its internal biological processes and its movements. The body constantly uses its internal stores of Qi, and it is essential to maintain a balance by replenishing them. QiGong is dedicated to that purpose.

Receiving external Qi

QiGong exercises gather fresh Qi from the external world and direct it into the body. Opening the arms to the sky invites energy from the sky to pour down through your body.

Imbibing fresh Qi

The body takes in Qi from the air, through breathing, from food, and during sleep. Good Qi is abundant in country areas where the air is fresh, and in natural, unadulterated food. It is scarce in built-up areas where the air quality is poor.

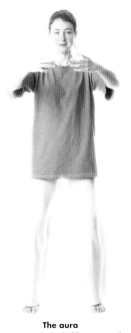

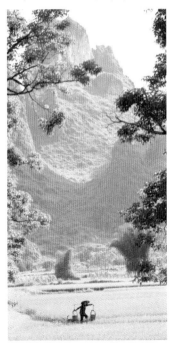

The aura

Qi permeates the body, filling every cell in every tissue. And it extends beyond it as the aura—a field of Qi electromagnetic energy that links internal and external Qi. Chinese scientists have detected the presence of Qi, but it is invisible to the eye. However, some people are able to see a person's aura.

Energy Flow

In traditional Chinese medicine, as in Ayurvedic and other Eastern medical systems, life energy or Qi is believed to be in motion in the body, flowing along meridians or channels called *mai* to reach all parts of it. These channels are invisible and do not appear on X rays or scans. They were discovered long ago by physicians practicing acupuncture, who detected 12 major meridians in the body. Each takes the name of an organ that it may pass through or is linked with in some other way. By *organ* the Chinese mean a physical structure—the heart, the lungs, the kidneys—and the associated parts of the body. To give an example, the lung meridians begin at the lungs, but the Chinese organ *Lung* includes the nose, the nasal passages, and the trachea. The lung meridian controls the entire process of breathing. In addition, each organ has functions that affect the mind and spirit. So the Lung, which receives Qi from outside the body, provides inspiration and a sense of meaning in life.

Acupressure and QiGong

The pathways the meridians follow around the body sometimes plunge deep beneath its surface and pass through organs. Where a pathway rises to just beneath the skin surface it can be treated by acupuncture. Along the superficial pathways of each meridian are located 365 acupuncture points, which can be stimulated by pressure from a needle. These points may also be stimulated manually, so they may also be called acupressure points.

Acupressure is involved in some QiGong exercises. For example, the fingers press the lung acupressure points in Gathering I on pages 130–131. The body is said to be in balance only when Qi can flow unimpeded along all meridians. A major aim of all QiGong exercises is to stimulate the flow of Qi along the meridians, regulating its flow rate, clearing blockages, releasing stale Qi into the external world, and opening the meridians to allow new Qi to enter from inside the body—released from the internal organs—and outside it.

The meridians

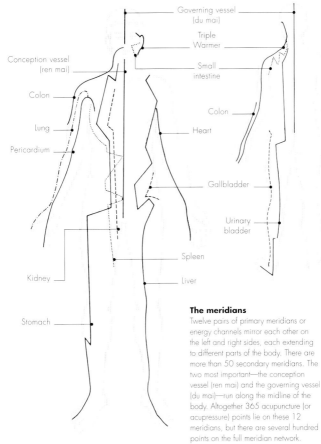

Governing vessel (du mai)

Triple Warmer

Small intestine

Conception vessel (ren mai)

Colon

Lung

Pericardium

Colon

Heart

Gallbladder

Urinary bladder

Kidney

Spleen

Liver

Stomach

The meridians

Twelve pairs of primary meridians or energy channels mirror each other on the left and right sides, each extending to different parts of the body. There are more than 50 secondary meridians. The two most important—the conception vessel (ren mai) and the governing vessel (du mai)—run along the midline of the body. Altogether 365 acupuncture (or acupressure) points lie on these 12 meridians, but there are several hundred points on the full meridian network.

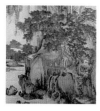

Contemplating energy
The concept of Qi was a major concern of Daoist sages, who retreated to remote places to meditate on nature.

ENERGY CENTERS

Spaced along the du mai meridian from the spine to the top of the head, are seven vortices of concentrated Qi. They correspond to the body's main plexes or networks of major nerves—the chung wan lies over the solar plexus—but their existence has not been proved. Each energy center also corresponds with endocrine glands, which release hormones directly into the blood. For example, the yin dang center in the forehead corresponds with the pineal gland, which produces melatonin and affects the cycle of sleep and wakefulness. QiGong movements stimulate one or more energy centers, and this helps regulate the flow of energy through the body, promoting healing. Each energy center is linked with emotions—so stimulating the heart center may improve mood and outlook. QiGong harnesses the healing power of movement to unblock feeling, ease physical disorders and pain, and increase awareness.

The primary energy centers
The illustration opposite shows the positions of the seven primary energy centers. The first, the hui yin, is the lowest, located at the base of the spine and the seventh, the pai hui, lies over the anterior fontanelle—the position of the soft spot at the top of a newborn baby's skull.

7 Pai hui: crown center
Location: cerebral cortex
Gland: pituitary
Associated body part: brain
Qualities: inspiration,
ideas, knowledge, wisdom

6 Yin dang: upper dantian, third
eye, or brow center
Location: middle of forehead
Gland: pineal
Body parts: eyes and brain
Qualities: visualization, symbolism,
dreaming, intuition, understanding

5 Hsuan chi:
throat center
Location: throat at
pharyngeal plexus
Glands: thyroid and
parathyroid
Body parts: throat,
neck, shoulders, ears,
nose, lungs
Qualities: expression of
feeling, communication

4 Middle dantian:
heart center
Location: between
shoulder blades/
center of chest
Gland: thymus
Body parts: heart,
lungs, arms, hands
Qualities: balance,
honesty, passion,
compassion, love
Element: air

3 Chung Wan: solar
plexus center
Location: solar plexus
Glands: adrenals,
pancreas
Body parts: stomach,
spleen, liver, muscles
Qualities: self-worth
and confidence
Element: fire

2 Lower dantian:
sacral center
Location: about 3 inches
(7 centimeters) below navel
Gland: ovaries
Body parts: kidneys, womb,
small intestine, bladder
Qualities: central gatherer
and distributor, strong
emotion, flow and change
Element: water

1 Hui yin: base or root center
Location: sacrum, lower pelvis
Gland: testicles
Body parts: sexual organs,
colon, legs, feet, bones
Qualities: sexual urge,
reproduction, survival
Element: Earth

Secondary Energy Gateways

Supplementing the body's seven primary energy centers shown on pages 30–31 are a number of secondary energy centers. When activated by QiGong movements, these secondary centers act as gateways for external energy to be absorbed into the body and to circulate within it, and for internal energy to pass out into the external world.

Activating the joints

Several secondary centers cluster around the principal movable joints. A joint is a point where two or more bones meet, and there are many different types. The junctions between most bones in the skull are immovable, and the joints of the spine and the pelvis have just a limited range of movement. Dynamic QiGong postures exercise the freely movable joints, and these movements activate secondary meridians and energy gateways associated with them.

Joints of the spine

The spine has 33 bones or vertebrae and three types of joint. The atlas and axis at the top have movable joints, which allow the head to nod and shake. Cervical, thoracic, and lumbar vertebrae are separated by disks of cartilage, which give more limited movement. The shield-shaped sacrum and the coccyx or tail bone consist of fused bones and are normally immobile, except during pregnancy. QiGong exercises stimulate the spine's main energy gateway, the ming men on the second lumbar vertebra.

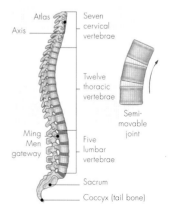

Atlas

Axis

Seven cervical vertebrae

Twelve thoracic vertebrae

Semi-movable joint

Ming Men gateway

Five lumbar vertebrae

Sacrum

Coccyx (tail bone)

Maintaining mobility

QiGong movements keep the joints mobile, preventing degenerative diseases from taking hold. Concentrating the mind on the part of the body being moved—on rotating the spine, for instance, or pressing the foot into the ground—activates the secondary energy centers associated with it.

Feng chi gateway. Stimulation eases head and neck pain

The elbow, shoulder, and hip joints are the sites of clusters of several energy centers.

Ming Men—the Gateway of Life—is an important energy center on the du mai meridian. Stimulation boosts energy flow along the spine.

Laogong points in the palms, just below the middle fingers, attract external energy when the palms are open.

Yongquan

Yongquan gateway

Earth energy enters the body through these gateways in the center of each forefoot and rises up the legs to the dantian.

Yongquan

PRINCIPLES AND POLARITIES

A fundamental principle of Chinese philosophy is the concept of yin and yang, the forces of dark and light, of change and harmony. Yin is seen as possessing the qualities of darkness and earth—it is soft and inward-looking. Yang is the opposite, it is the force of light and the sky—outward-looking and hard. Life may be seen as a search for equilibrium between the two, a perpetual changing from yin to yang and to yin again. Everything in the universe has yin or yang qualities, even the parts of the human body. Some meridians that channel Qi through the body are yang and are guided by the du mai or governing vessel, which travels up the spine. The ren mai or conception vessel, which travels up the front of the body, directs yin meridians. Polarities like yin and yang, soft and hard, open and closed, are reflected in QiGong exercises.

Full and empty

Stepping on page 166 involves emptying your weight from one side of the body to fill the other. As you step with your left foot, your weight flows out of your right leg and foot, pouring into your left leg as the foot touches the ground.

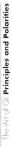

Ancient symbols

The ancient Chinese symbol for yin and yang is now widely recognized in the West. It represents the attainment of perfect equilibrium, yet it contains the seeds of perpetual change.

Standing Posture

QiGong seeks to make the most of the upright human stance, feet on the ground, head in the sky. It encourages correct alignment with the downward fall of gravity—a manifestation of cosmic energy. Like the trunk of a tree the spine grows upward, lifting the head toward the sky and the energy pouring down from the cosmos. It also links legs and feet to earth, enabling energy to rise through the yongquan gateway (see page 33).

Basic stance

The standing posture illustrated opposite is the basis of all QiGong exercises. When you are standing correctly you feel lifted from above and anchored from below, Earthed through your legs and feet, and held upright by the solidity of your spine. Begin by planting your feet hip-width apart, heels and toes aligned, and centering your weight: rock backward and forward, gradually making the rocking movement smaller and smaller until you find the center of each foot, then check that your weight is not pressing your feet toward the inside or outside edges. It needs to fall on the centerline of each foot.

Work up from the feet, first bending your knees slightly, then aligning your pelvis so your buttocks do not flatten nor stick out. Stretch the bones at the base of your pelvis—the bones you sit on—down toward the floor. This tucks your lower back in. While you are doing this, do not let your abdomen tighten. Consciously relax the muscles of your abdomen from your pelvis up to your chest. Relax your shoulders by lifting them high and dropping them. The position in which they fall is the natural one, so hold them there and do not let them hunch forward so your spine humps, or press back, so your chest sticks out.

Finally, lift your spine from the sacrum at the back of the pelvis to the atlas at the top, and lift the crown of your head toward the sky. Breathe normally, and remain relaxed. Standing like this sometimes feels awkward at first because we all develop poor postural habits. Practice until it is second nature.

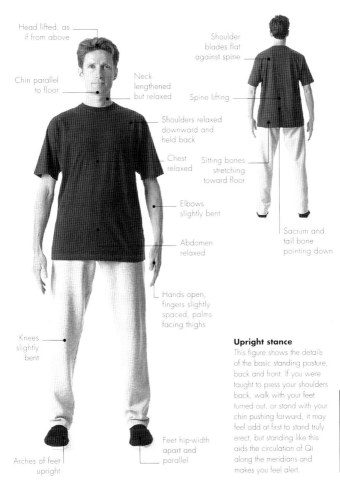

Head lifted, as if from above

Chin parallel to floor

Neck lengthened but relaxed

Shoulders relaxed downward and held back

Chest relaxed

Elbows slightly bent

Abdomen relaxed

Hands open, fingers slightly spaced, palms facing thighs

Knees slightly bent

Arches of feet upright

Feet hip-width apart and parallel

Shoulder blades flat against spine

Spine lifting

Sitting bones stretching toward floor

Sacrum and tail bone pointing down

Upright stance

This figure shows the details of the basic standing posture, back and front. If you were taught to press your shoulders back, walk with your feet turned out, or stand with your chin pushing forward, it may feel odd at first to stand truly erect, but standing like this aids the circulation of Qi along the meridians and makes you feel alert.

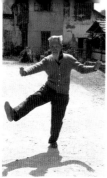

Any time, any place
The Chinese practice in open places where fresh air will clear the Qi fields of spent energy and replenish them with healthy Qi.

THE BREATH

Breathing links the human body and spirit with the external world. Breathing in is a yin action, which draws in new Qi from the external world to replace energy lost; breathing out expels stale Qi. Breathing in nourishes the body, since oxygen and other gases pass from the lungs into the bloodstream and are carried to the tissues. There they are absorbed as nutrients by cells, fueling the body processes. Breathing out clears and cleanses. Stale, used, internal Qi is breathed out, while air depleted of oxygen, but rich in carbon dioxide, nitrogen, and other gases the body no longer needs, is released. City air is now commonly high in pollutants and low in oxygen and Qi. If you live in a city, do not add to the pollution by driving a car. It is better to cycle and to walk, and to get out of the city as often as you can to the countryside, where breathing less polluted air will make you feel healthier.

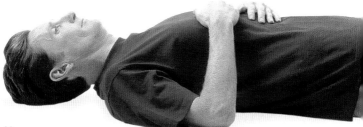

Opening the lungs

QiGong exercises in which you raise your arms above your head and stretch upward open the lungs. There are several in the form sequence in Chapter 4: this photograph shows step 1 of Awaken the Spine on page 98.

Deepening the breath

Lie on the floor with your head, spine, and feet in line, your legs together. Relax, let your feet fall open, and rest your hands on your lower ribs. Breathe normally and notice whether your ribs rise and fall with your breathing. Are you breathing through your mouth or your nose? Now take a longer, slower in-breath through the nose, then breathe out through the nose just as slowly. Your ribs should rise and fall more noticeably. Continue breathing deeply to a slow rhythm for two minutes or more.

Breathing and Exercise

Some historians believe QiGong originated when people learned to make different sounds with the breath, and that it first developed as breathing exercises. Today, there are advanced QiGong techniques that involve making sounds with different qualities while concentrating the mind on a desired healing effect.

Breathing is only partly under your control. Much of it is involuntary and the unconscious adapts it automatically to changing circumstances. It is therefore a mistake for beginners to focus too hard on breathing when practicing QiGong. There are no complex rules to follow. Just breathe normally and your breath will adjust to the pace and rhythm of the exercise. If you get out of breath or find yourself thinking about breathing, your breathing rhythm may be out of sync. People who live stressful lives sometimes develop hyperventilation—a habit of shallow breathing—as a response. Breathing is a way of taking in the Qi you need to work through the exercises without tiring, and if your breathing is superficial or irregular, you may need to practice deep rhythmic breathing (see pages 42–43).

Useful guidelines

There is one useful rule of thumb that applies to breathing while exercising: breathe out on exertion. For example, breathe in while lifting your arms, but breathe out while bending forward in Pressing to Earth on pages 102–103. Occasionally, where appropriate, an instruction is given on breathing during a particular exercise in the form.

In the words of Dr. Chi Chiang-tao, a Chinese teacher of taijiquan (t'ai chi ch'uan) who taught widely in the West: let the breath harmonize as you learn the moves. This is invaluable advice, because trying to make the breath fit the moves can be stressful, and this may impede the flow of Qi. Many beginners try too hard and so breathe forcefully, which has the same effect. It is best to feel your way, pausing when you are familiar with a movement to think about how your breath fits in with it.

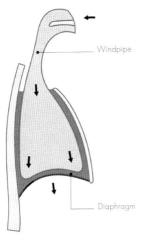

Windpipe

Diaphragm

Windpipe

Diaphragm

What happens when you breathe

Breathing happens because your lungs, ribs, and abdominal muscles work together to pump air in and out.

In-breath

As you breathe in, the large, flat muscle called the diaphragm, which stretches like a sheet across your lower chest, contracts and flattens, and the intercostal muscles, which fill the spaces between the ribs, relax. This pulls the ribcage out and down, and the expansion pulls air through the nose, down the windpipe and into your lungs.

Out-breath

Oxygen molecules in the air you breathe pass through the lung walls into surrounding blood vessels, and carbon dioxide molecules from used air pass from the blood into the lungs. The diaphragm relaxes, becoming dome-shaped, and pushes against the ribcage, and the intercostal muscles tighten. As a result, the volume of the chest decreases and the lungs deflate, squeezing air into the windpipe and out through the nose.

ABDOMINAL BREATHING

Breathing is a way of managing energy, so learning to control the breath is thought to have therapeutic benefits. Many QiGong masters have trained themselves to breathe more efficiently, inhaling more deeply, yet less often, and using less air than is normal. The breathing techniques they practice may be considered advanced, however. Beginners need to breathe naturally as shown on pages 40–41, but it can be helpful to beginners to learn abdominal breathing. This is considered especially important in QiGong since it increases energy by storing Qi at the dantian. Most adults breathe using just the chest, but QiGong teaches that it is natural to involve the abdomen as well as the chest. Abdominal breathing is thought to increase the therapeutic value of QiGong exercises. However, breathing is a semiconscious activity and it can be hard to learn to breathe in a different way. The exercises opposite are designed to help you learn, but you may need to practice regularly for weeks before it begins to feel natural. Use it in your practice only when you feel ready.

Awareness-raising

This is an elementary exercise intended to raise awareness of abdominal breathing, rather than a training exercise. In time, however, the movements of your abdomen will begin to adjust to the rhythm created by the pressure of your hand.

1 *Stand in the basic posture shown on page 37, then place one hand on your lower abdomen with the palm over the navel and the other over the dantian energy center 3 inches (7 centimeters) below it. Breathe normally for two minutes to check whether your abdomen rises and falls in time with your breath.*

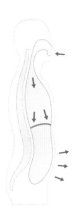

2 Breathe in deeply while thinking of your diaphragm relaxing and flattening, increasing the volume of the lungs and pressing down on the organs of your abdomen. As you breathe out, visualize the diaphragm contracting and becoming dome-shaped, pushing up against the lungs and decreasing the volume of air in them, but releasing its pressure on the abdomen.

3 Continue breathing fairly deeply while visualizing the movements of the diaphragm, and as you breathe out, gently press the abdomen in, releasing the pressure as you breathe in. Do this for up to two minutes at first, gradually increasing the length of time as you practice.

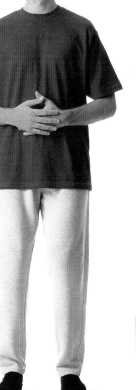

Breathing and Relaxation

When you think about the way you breathe during the exercise on pages 42–43, you may realize that you tighten up at the front as you breathe in and out. In fact, this is a common way of responding to stress: tightening the abdominal muscles feels like armoring yourself against negative feelings when you are under attack. However, squeezing the abdominals impedes the breathing a little, and it worsens tension.

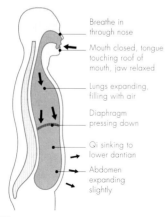

Breathe in through nose

Mouth closed, tongue touching roof of mouth, jaw relaxed

Lungs expanding, filling with air

Diaphragm pressing down

Qi sinking to lower dantian

Abdomen expanding slightly

Learning to relax is an important part of QiGong, and a good way of beginning is to relax all the muscles involved in breathing: the neck and throat, the shoulders, the chest, and the abdomen. Focusing the mind on the dantian when you are standing still, and on the movements during the dynamic exercises, helps you remain relaxed.

Learning to relax

Simple breathing exercises like those on pages 38–39 and 42–43 are a good way of practicing relaxation. One of the most effective ways of relieving tension instantly is to practice deep breathing with the emphasis on the out-breath: breathe in, but breathe out for longer. As you breathe out, relax all the muscles of your abdomen from the chest to the groin. This is a good thing to do in a tense situation: stop, take

Practising abdominal breathing
Focus your mind on the lower dantian and breathe into it while relaxing your body. Your shoulders do not rise, and as you breathe in the Qi descends to the lower dantian to be stored. Keep your abdomen relaxed as you breathe out and a reservoir of Qi remains there.

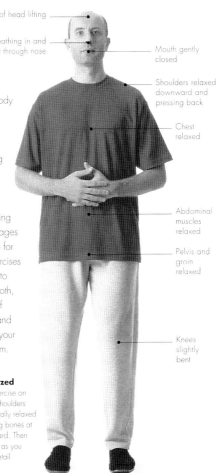

Top of head lifting

Breathing in and out through nose

Mouth gently closed

Shoulders relaxed downward and pressing back

Chest relaxed

Abdominal muscles relaxed

Pelvis and groin relaxed

Knees slightly bent

a few deep breaths, relax, and continue. Mind and body always work together, so you cannot relax fully without relaxing mind as well as muscles. Visualizing Qi residing in the dantian helps relax the muscles involved in breathing.

The exercises in breathing and relaxation on these pages make a good preparation for the dynamic QiGong exercises and the form. It is difficult to achieve the graceful, smooth, and flowing movements of QiGong if there is stress and tension in your mind and your body when you make them.

Awareness-raising analyzed

Begin the awareness-raising exercise on pages 41–42 by raising your shoulders and letting them fall into a naturally relaxed position and stretching the sitting bones at the base of your pelvis downward. Then keeping your shoulders relaxed as you breathe, check through each detail pinpointed on this figure.

DYNAMIC QIGONG

The breathing exercises on the last few pages and the basic stance on pages 36–37 are static forms of QiGong. Static exercises are designed to open the body's energy centers and to build internal power through posture and concentration. There are many static postures in QiGong, performed sitting and lying down as well as standing. These are outnumbered, however, by a range of moving exercises, known as dynamic QiGong. The movements are designed to be performed as sequences, and they often imitate the way birds and animals move. Chapter 4 introduces a sequence of 128 exercises based on the movements of the crane. QiGong movements are designed to help the body flow, internally and externally.

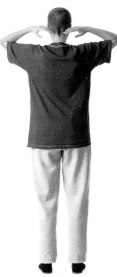

In the exercises, the whole body merges smoothly from one slow, graceful movement into another, as if powered by relaxation rather than by effort. Such light, fluid movements can only be achieved with strong, elastic joints and muscles, plus great concentration. These take time and dedicated practice to achieve, but bring immediate rewards in the form of greater poise and confidence in moving, better concentration, and a sense of well-being.

Moving exercises

QiGong has many classic movements that do not appear in the White Crane form in Part 4. Clearing the aura is one. In step 1 you lift your hands to stimulate the nerves at the base of the skull.

Clearing the aura

In step 2 you bend forward from the hips, sweeping your hands to your feet to rest them, palms facing the floor, just above your insteps. This movement clears stale Qi from your aura.

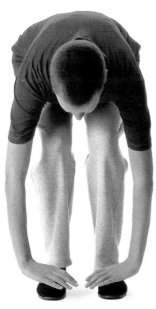

Freestyle movement

Do not be afraid to allow the body to move freely using movements you know from practicing the form as shown above. It gives a sense of balance and focus, and teaches coordination.

Muscles and Movement

One of the objectives of QiGong is to restore the body's natural elasticity. Movable joints become stiff and painful when they are not used, and in danger of developing degenerative disease. QiGong exercises all the joints with slow, gentle movements so that after practice you feel as if your joints have been oiled.

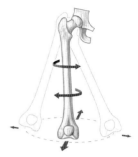

The mobile hip joint

During a normal working day the hip joint may do little more than lift or lower, but to remain mobile, it needs to be exercised through its extraordinary range of movement two or three times a week.

Developing elasticity

QiGong movements are light and flowing, but they make the muscles work, building strength and stamina. They stretch and strengthen all the skeletal muscles—those attached by tendons to bones—and keep the tendons supple. They do not impose heavy weight burdens, however. Weight lifting causes muscles to increase in bulk through contraction, while QiGong stretches muscles and tendons out, gradually building up their resistance. The result is greater elasticity plus exceptional power and strength. Holding the arms at shoulder height to perfect the waving motion of Undulating Arms on pages 86–93 develops the muscular strength of a weight lifter with the delicacy of movement of a dancer.

Many people complain of clumsiness and lack of coordination. QiGong involves the mind in every movement, encouraging you to focus your attention on the flow of Qi while you are moving, and this improves coordination. This process of converting thought to feeling is a central aspect of QiGong.

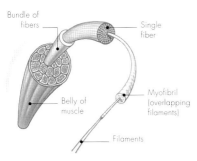

Muscle action

Muscles that move joints consist of bundles of long fibers, all running in the same direction. Each fiber consists of bands of filaments that overlap when the muscle is relaxed. When stimulated by a brain impulse traveling along a nerve, the filaments slide over each other, shortening the muscle fiber and so making the muscle contract.

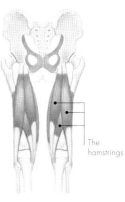

The hamstrings

Tendons attach muscles to bones. Some muscles, such as the three at the back of the thighs, have very long tendons. They are the hamstrings, and if they are not stretched regularly, they tighten, so that bending forward with the legs straight becomes very painful.

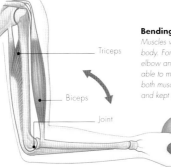

Bending and stretching

Muscles work in pairs to move joints to move the body. For example, the biceps muscle bends the elbow and the triceps muscle straightens it. To be able to move the joint smoothly, without jerking, both muscles need to be worked regularly and kept strong.

MIND PLAY

QiGong means "energy work" but it could equally be called "mind work" since Qi follows the lead of the mind. A major aim of QiGong is to control the mind in order to be able to guide and direct the Qi. But many beginners find the mental aspects of QiGong hard to master. If you have experienced the calm and sense of well-being that the physical exercises bring you, expect the mind exercises to bring similar benefits, and expect them to be fun. Visualizations are like children's games, which turn imagination into reality. Adults have to rediscover how to set the imagination free. The way to achieve this freedom is to practice exercises like those opposite. They may seem childish at first, but they help you discover your personal creativity, which may have been lost in the shouldering of adult responsibilities.

Think pink

If you find it hard to do visualization exercises, stop trying, and play games with your mind. The idea is to convert a thought into a feeling.

1 *Stand in the middle of a room, close your eyes, and visualize the room. Look at the floor and in your mind's eye watch it turn bright pink. Notice the shade of pink and watch the pink as it seeps toward your feet. Watch your shoes turn pink, and watch the pink creep up your legs and up your body, turning you the same bright shade.*

2 *Keeping your eyes closed, look at the pool of pink in which you stand and ask yourself how you feel about it. What effect does the shade of pink have on you? How do you feel about being bright pink from head to toe? Think pink for as long as you like, exploring aspects of your new pink status. Then open your eyes.*

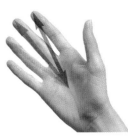

Drawing connections

1 Stand with your hands by your sides, then raise one hand to eye level, palm facing you. Look at the middle of your palm and imagine that a black dot appears there. Center your attention on it, then pull it out with your eyes and carefully draw a black line up to the tip of your fourth finger, then draw it back to the center of your palm.

2 Repeat step 1, drawing a line from the center of your palm to the tip of your third finger and back. And as you slowly draw the line, visualize the line activating a flow of Qi to the fingertip and back to the palm.

3 Repeat step 2, drawing a line to the tip of your middle finger and back to the palm, watching the Qi flow up to the fingertip as you slowly draw the line with your eyes. As the line moves and the Qi flows, do you notice any sensation on the surface of your hand?

4 Repeat step 2, this time drawing a line to the tip of your index finger and back to the palm. Concentrate on feeling the Qi move as you slowly draw the line to the fingertip. Detecting just the subtlest flutter of sensation is evidence that your thought has become feeling and your mind is leading your Qi.

Awareness and Concentration

Unlike almost all movements in sports, many QiGong movements have no obvious purpose—there is no ball to hit or kick. You create the ball through visualization and imagine yourself catching and throwing it. Visualization helps you understand how you need to move and why. It makes the exercises work and the movements more interesting.

Cultivating awareness

The mind has a central role in all QiGong exercises. In fact the movements you make with your body are only half of what is happening. The aim of every exercise is to bring new energy to the body, to store it or to send it where it is needed, and it is awareness of this energy that brings these movements about. As your body moves, your mind moves too, now directing your awareness to activate and guide the flow of Qi along a rising arm, now focusing on Qi radiating outward

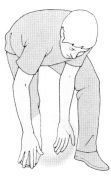

Bringing the mind into play
Awareness adds a dimension to QiGong exercises which makes the movements easier and fun to do. For example, making the correct arm movements in Spinning Ball on pages 106–107 is much easier if you visualize yourself spinning a ball between your hands.

from a palm, now concentrating on Earth energy rising from beneath a foot. Without this awareness, the energy may not flow, or radiate, or rise.

It takes concentration to coordinate the movements of mind and body, and to make energy flow. Being able to turn thought into feeling as shown on pages 50–51 trains the concentration. Trying to force the mind to concentrate by imagining energy moving along an arm, back to the shoulder, then back to a hand requires too great an effort. It is easier to visualize the energy as a wave washing back and forth along your arm, since it puts the thought in touch with a feeling.

Achieving the impossible

Mental awareness is the essence of QiGong. There are reports of injured and disabled people bringing about remarkable physical healing through QiGong by learning to direct their healing energy to the places in their body where it could cause change. Concentrating the awareness is the self-healing technique that brings this change about. And visualization brings a bonus in that it leads to self-knowledge and the ability to realize seemingly unattainable goals.

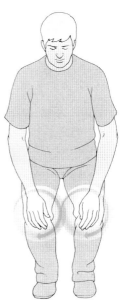

Healing hands

Sit on a chair and put your hands on your knees. Feel the warm Qi from your hands pass through your palms into your knees. Qi is good, healing energy, which may be used to bring relief to other people simply by touching them with your palm.

WARM UP

Chapter 3 introduces some important and fundamental QiGong exercises for body and mind. ✎ Some, like Earth Wash on pages 70–71 and the warm-up exercises on pages 58–59 and 62–63, are dynamic or moving exercises, while others, such as Standing Like a Pillar on pages 66–67, are static or quiescent exercises. ✎ The following pages present them all as a preparation for the collection of movements known as the form, White Crane, which follows in Chapter 4, but like all QiGong exercises, these may also be carried out independently. The rhythmic, repetitive movements of Earth Wash are an excellent antidote to stress, for example. ✎ All QiGong exercises seek to develop Qi or life energy (see pages 26–27) and the chapter ends by defining the pathways that Qi follows around the body.

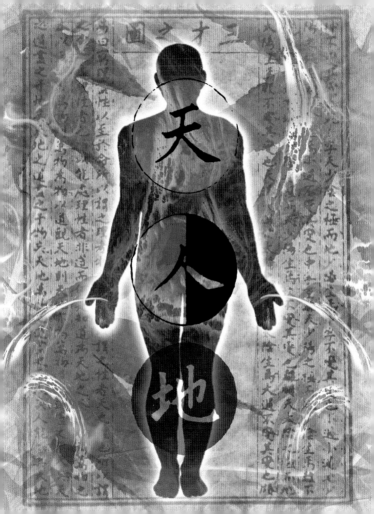

Loosening Up

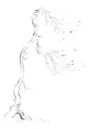

Blowing in the wind

Imagine the branches of a tree blowing in wind and imitate its movements with your trunk, your arms, and your head. Keep your feet on the ground and move from the hips.

Although QiGong is not a sport, a few minutes' general warm up is beneficial before performing any activity. Loosening-up movements stretch muscles and tendons, making them more elastic for when you begin the QiGong exercises. It is known that in high-impact sports, warming up makes the muscles less susceptible to injury. Older people are particularly prone to strain from exercising without a gentle warm up. The warm-up exercises on pages 58–59 and 62–63 rehearse some of the movements you will be making when you start the form, and this prepares you mentally, so that your movements are more coordinated and smoother.

Warming up the mind

Little scientific research has been done on warming up and there is as yet no hard experimental proof that warm up improves physical performance, but its psychological benefits are widely accepted. A gradual, brief warm up

Benefits of Warming Up

Physiologists believe gentle warm-up exercises may benefit the body in the following ways:

• Higher core body temperatures may speed nerve impulses traveling along nerve fibers and so increase the response time of muscles to commands from the brain

• The resistance to movement of structures inside the muscles may be lowered

• Higher core body temperatures may increase the amount of oxygen available to the muscles

• Higher temperatures in the muscles cause the blood vessels serving them to widen, so increasing the amount of blood, and therefore of oxygen and other nutrients to the body tissues.

that increases body and muscle temperature just before practice will improve your confidence and outlook.

Loosen your mind as well as your body by trying the mental exercises on these two pages. While stretching your imagination they will help you develop spontaneity and fluidity in movement without any strain. You may also enjoy making up your own program of movements. Put on some music and move in time to it, improvising.

Floating under water

Move as if you were an underwater plant rooted in a riverbed, your fronds moving gently with the current.

Program

You can improvise exercises and move freely to warm up, but if you prefer to have a program to follow, this one makes a good 10-minute introduction to the form in Chapter 4. Exercise to music if you wish.

1 Shakeout (see page 58)	2 minutes
2 Head circles (see page 59)	30 seconds
3 Leg swings (see page 62)	1 minute
4 Clapping (see page 211)	30 seconds
5 Sunrise (see page 63)	2 minutes
6 Sunset (see page 63)	2 minutes
7 Earth Wash (see pages 70–71)	2 minutes

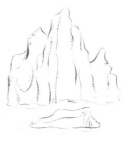

Ocean journey

Now float like an iceberg moving majestically on the surface of the ocean, towed by the currents and buffeted by waves.

WARM-UP EXERCISES: 1

The following set of short exercise routines make an excellent warm-up sequence before beginning the form. They move the whole body from head to toe, stretching muscles and joints and stimulating the nervous system and the circulation of the blood, the lymph, and Qi. The exercises shown on these two pages rotate the head, neck, and trunk, and stretch and move the limbs. Those on pages 62–63 concentrate on whole-body movements. Their combined effect is to relax and to energize.

Shakeout

Shaking your whole body from the feet up while bending and straightening your legs will warm you up on a cold day. This is a great exercise to do to music.

1 Stand with your feet hip-width apart. Start by lifting each leg in turn and shaking first the foot, then the whole leg.

2 Hold both arms a few inches from your body and shake your hands from the wrists, then your arms from the shoulders.

3 With heels and toes touching the ground, shake your whole body up to the head, then continue shaking for a minute or more while bending and straightening your legs. Then rest.

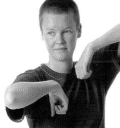

Conductor

Stand with your feet hip-width apart, bend your elbows, placing your fingers on your shoulder joint, and move your elbows from the sides to the front. Now imagine an orchestra ranged in front of you and conduct it, using your elbows, for about 30 seconds. Then write your first name with each elbow in turn.

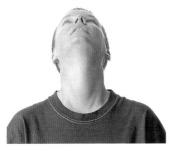

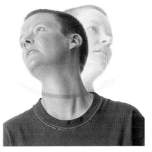

Neck stretches

This exercise is good for relieving an aching neck. Before you begin to move, lift your shoulders and let them fall naturally. Keep your back and shoulders relaxed and straight throughout. Breathe normally.

1 Stand upright with your feet less than hip-width apart and your hands by your sides. Breathe normally. Leading with your eyes, turn your head slowly as far right as you can, then as far to the left. Repeat twice, then turn to face forward.

2 Now lift your head up and tilt it back, letting your mouth open as you look as far behind you as you can. Then slowly lift your head and drop it forwards until your chin touches your chest. Repeat twice, then raise your head to look forward.

Head circles

Continue in the same position as for Neck Stretches. Move your head slowly and smoothly, continuing to breathe normally. If you feel dizzy at any stage, stop immediately.

1 Next, draw as large a circle as you can in the air by circling your chin clockwise. Repeat twice, then circle your chin counterclockwise three times.

2 When you have completed the first stage, stand still for about a minute with your eyes closed.

Heaven and Earth

In the past, the Chinese masters of QiGong closely observed the body and the way it moves, and searched for ways of standing and moving that would best support its structure and maintain its mobility and flexibility through a long life. Static or quiescent QiGong exercises emphasize posture. To do its job of holding the body upright, the spine must always be aligned naturally, but this does not mean straight, for the bones of the spine form three natural curves. The standing postures stretch each one strongly up from the sacrum at its base to the atlas on which the skull rests.

The dynamic exercises are based on the knowledge that if the joints of the spine and the limbs are to remain mobile into old age they need regular movement throughout life. A full sequence of QiGong exercises like that in Chapter 4 gently exercises every one of the body's movable joints.

Gate of heaven

Cosmic energy enters the body through the pai hui gateway in the crown. It lies at the convergence of eight meridians—three on the left side and three on the right which originate in the feet, plus the liver meridian and the governing vessel.

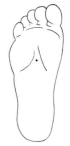

Gateway to the Earth

Earth energy enters the body through the gateway in the feet called the yongquan. The yongquan is located in the center of each forefoot.

Posture and movement

QiGong links posture and movement with the concepts of the ancient Daoists, who saw the upright human body, feet on the ground, head in the sky, as a natural conductor of energy between the Earth and the cosmos. Through their exercises, they also sought to maintain and emphasize this natural alignment. So in QiGong exercises the body is firmly based—a concept called "grounding"— and its natural upward thrust, maintained by active muscles, is maximized, so the crown of the head stretches up to the heavens. By raising your arms to the sky and opening them, you invite the energy of the cosmos to pour down through your head and body. By stepping and standing you tap into the rich store of Earth energy, causing it to rise through your feet and to your head.

The following pages show you how QiGong puts the concepts of grounding and lifting to practical use in standing and in rhythmic movement. Practice them for a few minutes every day, and apply them in every aspect of your life.

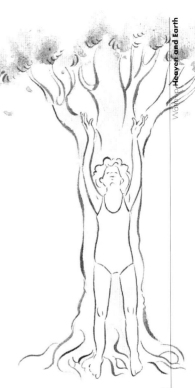

Root and trunk
The spine is a tree trunk that lifts you up to the heavens so that your hands may connect with the energy of the cosmos and attract it downward. When you stand and step, your feet send roots into the Earth, tapping into a well of nourishing Earth energy.

WARM-UP EXERCISES: 2

Feel you can be spontaneous about warming up. Begin by working through all the movable joints of your body—neck, shoulders, elbows, wrists, hips, fingers, knees, and just loosen them up—move them back, forward, up, down, and around, any way you can think of. Lift each leg in turn and see how many ways you can think of to move it. These two pages focus on the spine and the lower body. Sunrise opens the lungs, deepens the breathing, and lifts the spirits. Sunset, its complementary, has a calming effect. Both are good exercises to finish a warm up before commencing the standing meditation at the start of the form.

Leg Swings

Loosen your hip and ankle joints with these leg swings. They are an excellent exercise for older people, helping to keep the hips mobile. If you find it hard to keep your balance while swinging your legs, support yourself with one hand against a wall or resting on a table or other piece of heavy furniture.

1 *Stand upright with your arms by your sides, lift your right leg, and swing it back and forth.*

2 *On a forward swing, point your toes forward, then on the next, point the toes up and lead with the heel.*

3 *Lower your right leg, transfer your weight to it, and repeat the exercise, swinging your left leg. Then lower your left leg and stand upright.*

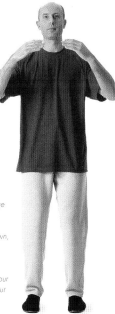

Sunrise

1 *Stand with your feet hip-width apart, hands by your sides, your knees relaxed. Slowly raise your hands to shoulder height, turning the palms toward you. Visualize sunlight filling your body, creating an aura around you, and raise both hands above your head. Straighten your arms up, lifting your face toward the sun.*

2 *Arc your hands down, opening your arms wide and lowering your head to face forward. Radiate goodwill. Center yourself, distributing your weight evenly on both feet, and lower your hands to your sides, then repeat steps 1 and 2.*

Sunset

1 *Stand with your feet hip-width apart, arms by your sides, knees relaxed. Arc your arms out to the sides and up in a large circle until the palms face each other above your head.*

2 *Bend your elbows and lower your hands, palms facing down, fingertips about 2 inches (5 centimeters) apart opposite your chin, then slowly move them down to the level of your navel.*

3 *Repeat steps 1 and 2 twice, imagining the sun setting as your hands sink, then rest them on the lower dantian. Straighten your legs; raise your left hand to the center of your chest, and rest.*

Preparation for QiGong Practice

Warming up is an important preparation for any exercise, even for the gentle movements of QiGong. Apart from the physical benefits, warming up relaxes you, and for QiGong to be effective it is essential to be relaxed. People are often tense at first, so they find it hard to concentrate on the visualizations and their movements are rather mechanical. You need to warm up for about five minutes even before practicing standing meditations. Since the form always begins with a standing meditation, complete the warm up and stand quietly for a few seconds. When you begin you will find your mind and your movements are more fluid.

Where to practice

QiGong requires little preparation—you can exercise anywhere—but choose as healthy a place as you can for your practice. The ideal is to find a place outdoors where the air is fresh, near

Guidelines for practice

TRY TO AVOID practising immediately after eating, or eating immediately after a QiGong session. Wait for half an hour before and after eating or drinking.

TRY TO FIND a few quiet minutes to let body and mind settle just before and just after a practice. QiGong masters recommend up to half an hour of quiet solitude after practice whenever this is possible, so do not rush off to meet other people immediately after completing the form.

TRY NOT TO interrupt QiGong sessions (even with a visit to the lavatory—try to find time during the half hour before or after practice). Put a "Do not disturb" notice on the door of your practice room, switch telephones over to an answering facility, switch off alarms.

DO NOT practice the form (White Crane QiGong on pages 78–177) when you are extremely tired—because of overwork, say. It is better to do a few warm-up exercises followed by some relaxing breathing and one or two calming movements, such as Earth Wash (see pages 70–71) for a few minutes, and then to rest and sleep.

TRY TO involve your whole self, mind and body, in every session of QiGong. Practising half-heartedly achieves little.

trees and water where it is replete
with life-giving Qi. However, this may
not be possible for most people, and it
is more important to practice regularly
than to practice surrounded by nature.
Whenever you are out in the wild,
taking the opportunity to do a few
QiGong exercises can be a wonderful
experience and can also benefit your
health. However, it is considered
unwise to practice QiGong in wind,
since it is said to dissipate internal
energy and to blow fresh Qi away.
If you live in a city, perhaps you can
exercise in a park or a garden. If you
have to hold your sessions indoors,
open the window for a while before
you begin to clear the air—or, if there
are fumes around, shut the window.

You do not need any equipment for
QiGong, other than a mat or a blanket
to lie on, nor any special clothing. It is
best to wear comfortable, loose-fitting
clothes and to practice in light shoes
with no heel.

STANDING LIKE A PILLAR

The next four pages are the first of several in the book that show a standing meditation, an exercise that combines the powers of body and mind to build energy. In Standing Like a Pillar, you use your mind to start your energy moving, although your body movements are minimal. This is achieved by focusing the mind on three of the seven major energy centers. Learning to involve the mind in physical exercise is an essential part of QiGong. These two pages focus on the physical aspects of this important exercise, and the two pages that follow explain the role of the mind.

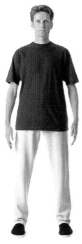

1 *Stand with your feet hip-width apart, your weight evenly distributed on the heels and soles of both feet, your shoulders relaxed, shoulder blades flat against your ribs, and your hands by your sides, palms turned toward your thighs.*

2 *Bend your knees slightly and raise your hands, turning the palms to an angle of about 45° to your body as you do so. Rest them slightly cupped opposite the lower dantian with the middle fingers about 2 inches (5 centimeters) apart, the fourth fingers closest to the body, and the index fingers uppermost. Allow your spine to lift your head toward the sky, and soften (relax) the crown of your head and the front of your body.*

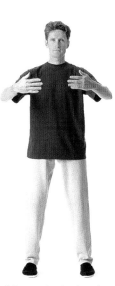

Third eye (upper dantian)

Heart center (middle dantian)

Sacral center (lower dantian)

3 Raise your hands in front of you level with your upper chest, palms facing inward, and move them together until the middle fingers are some 6 inches (15 centimeters) apart. Stand upright, firmly grounded, the top of your head lifting, and your shoulders, arms, and hands making a circle. Stand for up to 10 minutes, breathing into the lower dantian

Making connections

Standing meditations are a way of connecting with the major energy centers (see pages 30–31) and building energy there. You can hold your hands, palms facing, opposite the lower dantian as shown in step 2 in the exercise opposite; in line with the heart center as shown in step 3; or opposite the brow center or third eye, as shown above. You hold your arms in the chosen position for a few minutes while concentrating on building energy in that point. Your mind stimulates the flow of Qi at that energy center.

Activating the Mind

Standing Like a Pillar on pages 66–67 activates your Qi even though you stand perfectly still. To achieve this, you harness the powers of your mind and imagination. Begin in step 1 by focusing your mind on the lower dantian, the starting point for the circulation of life energy around the body. Close your eyes and visualize the energy as a pool filling with warm liquid gold, and as you lift your hands to the lower dantian in step 2, half-turn the palms outward to stop the golden Qi from spilling out of the pool.

Using your imagination

As the Qi rises up your spine, raise your hands with it up to your heart center to stimulate the energy flow there. Imagine a pillar rising up from the ground below your feet, through your outstretched arms and up into the heavens. Encircle the pillar with your arms, your fingers meeting on the far side of it, and hug it to your chest while remaining firmly grounded, your toes and heels touching on the floor. The pillar carries life-giving

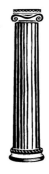

Hugging a pillar
Imagine you are standing before a pillar as you raise your hands in step 3 on page 67 and stretch your arms out wide as if you are going to embrace it. Imagine the feel of your arms and hands against the stone.

Qi up from the Earth's deep stores of energy and down from the cosmos to nourish you. Soften (relax) the energy gateways in your head and your feet.

Stand, absorbed in this meditation, for as long as you like. At first, you may return to the standing posture after two or three minutes, but as you perceive the value of the exercise you will find each meditation session lasting longer.

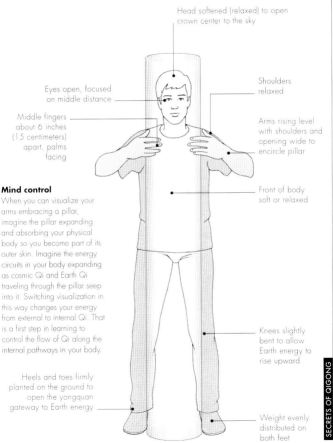

Head softened (relaxed) to open crown center to the sky

Shoulders relaxed

Eyes open, focused on middle distance

Arms rising level with shoulders and opening wide to encircle pillar

Middle fingers about 6 inches (15 centimeters) apart, palms facing

Mind control

When you can visualize your arms embracing a pillar, imagine the pillar expanding and absorbing your physical body so you become part of its outer skin. Imagine the energy circuits in your body expanding as cosmic Qi and Earth Qi traveling through the pillar seep into it. Switching visualization in this way changes your energy from external to internal Qi. That is a first step in learning to control the flow of Qi along the internal pathways in your body.

Front of body soft or relaxed

Knees slightly bent to allow Earth energy to rise upward

Heels and toes firmly planted on the ground to open the yongquan gateway to Earth energy

Weight evenly distributed on both feet

EARTH WASH

Like the static exercise on the last four pages, Earth Wash uses visualization, but it combines it with movement. Although it is a very simple introductory movement, it conveys the body/mind spirit of QiGong, for imagery powers the movements in every dynamic QiGong exercise. The benefits of this approach quickly become clear. You begin to feel more relaxed after just a minute or two of practice, and you sense your energy strengthening. This rhythmic, calming exercise is a marvelous antidote to frustration and tensions, a quick pick-me-up at stressful times.

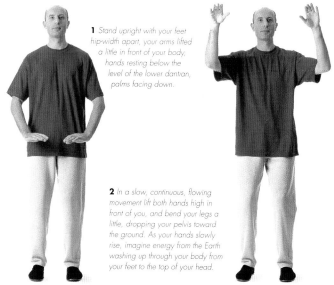

1 *Stand upright with your feet hip-width apart, your arms lifted a little in front of your body, hands resting below the level of the lower dantian, palms facing down.*

2 *In a slow, continuous, flowing movement lift both hands high in front of you, and bend your legs a little, dropping your pelvis toward the ground. As your hands slowly rise, imagine energy from the Earth washing up through your body from your feet to the top of your head.*

3 As your arms are rising level with the top of your head, begin to lower your arms slowly in a continuous, flowing movement, level with the lower dantian. At the same time, straighten your legs and lift your pelvis. As your hands float down, picture energy washing from the top of your head to your feet, and back into the Earth.

Repeat and rest

Repeat steps 2 and 3 over and over so that your arms rise and fall and your trunk falls and rises in a continuous, rhythmic movement. Continue for about two minutes—or longer if you enjoy the movement— then lower your hands to your sides, and rest in the standing posture.

Harnessing the Imagination

Standing at the beginning of Earth Wash on pages 70–71, your fingers pointing down, you feel in contact with the ground through your hands as well as your feet. You bend your knees, and as your spine drops, your hands come up. Then you reverse the movement. As your hands push down, the life energy in your palms, which just lifted from the Earth to the top of your head, washes down through your body and back to the ground.

Try to relax

Earth Wash puts you in practical touch with the principles of QiGong movement (see pages 46–49). Your arms need to flow smoothly, the downward movement following the upward lift without a break. Small movements of the muscles of your shoulder girdle power the raising and lowering of your arms. The more relaxed your shoulders, the more your arms and wrists will seem to float up, hands and fingers following, and then float

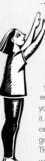

Sun-basking

Practise this static visualization exercise when you feel cold. If you can really imagine the warming effect of sunlight your whole body will feel warmed through in minutes.

While in the Standing Like a Pillar pose (see page 67), focus your mind on the crown energy center at the top of your head, and soften (relax) it. Raise your eyes to the ceiling and imagine you are gazing into bright sunlight. Think of the Sun's enveloping warmth, and imagine its rays descending toward you. Raise your hands toward the Sun, turning your palms outward, and imagine the Sun responding by pouring warm, golden Qi into your crown center and through your body to your feet. Feel the warmth of the Qi radiate outward, warming your body from within, bathing your limbs in its clear light.

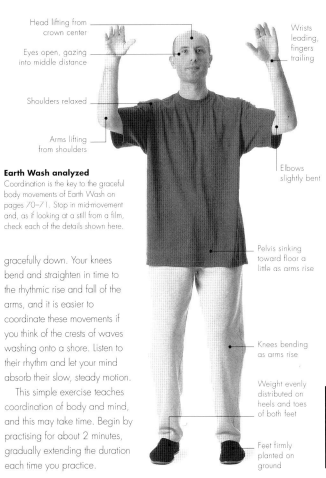

Head lifting from
crown center

Wrists
leading,
fingers
trailing

Eyes open, gazing
into middle distance

Shoulders relaxed

Arms lifting
from shoulders

Elbows
slightly bent

Earth Wash analyzed
Coordination is the key to the graceful
body movements of Earth Wash on
pages 70–71. Stop in mid-movement
and, as if looking at a still from a film,
check each of the details shown here.

Pelvis sinking
toward floor a
little as arms rise

gracefully down. Your knees
bend and straighten in time to
the rhythmic rise and fall of the
arms, and it is easier to
coordinate these movements if
you think of the crests of waves
washing onto a shore. Listen to
their rhythm and let your mind
absorb their slow, steady motion.

Knees bending
as arms rise

Weight evenly
distributed on
heels and toes
of both feet

This simple exercise teaches
coordination of body and mind,
and this may take time. Begin by
practising for about 2 minutes,
gradually extending the duration
each time you practice.

Feet firmly
planted on
ground

THE MICROCOSMIC ORBIT

Old manuscripts drawn up by Chinese physicians of the past show Qi traveling around the body along pathways called circuits, cycles, or orbits. Supreme among them is the heavenly cycle, which embraces several meridians. Through movement, breathing, and visualization, QiGong strengthens the circulation of Qi along the pathways. Beginners first learn to do this by activating the microcosmic orbit, sometimes called the small energy circuit because it follows just two meridians. To do this, you simply concentrate your mind on the lower dantian—Standing Like A Pillar (see pages 66–67) initiates the flow of Qi along this pathway. The next step is to stimulate a continuous flow around the circuit, and this involves following the route of the Qi in the mind. Each part of the White Crane form begins with a standing meditation to stimulate the flow of Qi around the microcosmic orbit. A strong energy flow around this circuit is considered of paramount importance by QiGong masters who believe it has a major role in preventing illnesses.

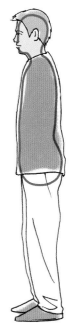

Energy circuits in the body

The microcosmic orbit is a natural energy circuit, the major pathway for the circulation of Qi in the upper body. It merges the two most important secondary meridians into a continuous orbit. One, the ren mai or conception vessel, begins at the perineum (the outer layer of tissue in the groin), rises up the trunk, into and through the neck, and terminates in the roof of the mouth. The second, the du mai or governing meridian, runs from the perineum up the spine, circulates around the head, before meeting the ren mai at the hard palate.

Switching on the circuit

Raising the arms in front and lowering them gently to the level of the dantian, as in Earth Wash, activates the circulation of Qi around the microcosmic orbit. It raises the Qi up the spine and brings it down the front of the body to the lower dantian.

Meridian Maintenance

Do this exercise often to activate and clear the meridians forming the microcosmic orbit.

1 Stimulate the microcosmic orbit by breathing into the lower dantian while concentrating Qi on gathering and building there: imagine a lake filling with water.

2 When the lake is full, move your mind's eye down toward the groin, feeling water from the lake wash through your skin from the living cells of the epidermis to the dead cell layer at the surface, and through the perineum (the outer tissues of the groin) and flow up your spine and around your skull. From the top of your head it washes through your face to the roof of your mouth, through your tongue, jaw, chin, and throat, and down your trunk to the lower dantian.

3 Repeat step 2 for two minutes at first, building up to three. Eventually, you might visualize this circuit for up to ten minutes.

Activating Energy Circuits

You may have to work at freeing your mind to visualize energy circulating around your body, but it is worth making the mental effort because the ability to visualize is a key technique that will enable you to relax at will.

Once you can send your imagination in any direction, you need to feel the energy circulate. Very often, physical tension blocks sensation, so it is important to practice relaxing the front of your body. This will help you sense the movement of Qi at the lower dantian. It is aided by rhythmic breathing, prolonging the out-breaths, which relaxes the muscles of the abdomen. This sets the pump in motion that sends Qi rising up your spine on its journey round the microcosmic orbit.

Detecting moving energy

Some people first sense the microcosmic energy move at the base of the spine. Others find they quickly notice signs of moving Qi—a warm feeling at the lower dantian, just below the navel, sensations of cold, lights before the eyes, or tingling feelings.

Being able to visualize and feel energy flow along the microcosmic orbit are early steps in learning to direct your mind and your Qi along any meridian to any part of your body at any time. Achieving this skill takes practice, and for this purpose the dantian pathways have been created. Following these two pathways with the mind as shown in the exercises on these pages trains you to link your mind with your Qi.

Focusing on each of the dantian pathways activates the three dantian energy centers (see pages 30–31). The lower circuit activates the lower dantian and the yongquan energy gateway in each foot, and helps stimulate a flow of Qi in the legs. It balances the energies of the lower body and so improves core stability, which in QiGong is called grounding or Earthing (see page 56). The upper circuit activates the laogong energy points in the palms, the yin dang or third eye center in the brow, and the heart center. It generates expansive feeling and warm spirit, and it balances the energies of the upper body.

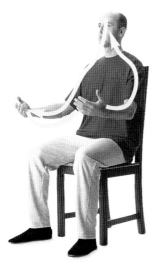

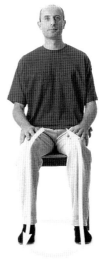

Upper dantian pathway

This circuit begins at the laogong center in the left palm and travels up the arm to the shoulder, up the neck and through the left temple to the yin dang or third eye in the center of the brow. It then moves down the right side of the body to the right palm.

1 *Sit on a chair and raise your hands in front of your chest, palms up. Imagine a ball of golden light in the center of your left palm and follow it along an illuminated pathway to the third eye, where you see a silver ball of light.*

2 *Move your mind's eye down through the right temple to the neck, along the right shoulder and down the arm toward a golden light in the right palm. Then arc across to the left hand and continue the circuit. This visualization should last 3–5 minutes at first, building up to 15 minutes.*

Lower dantian pathway

This circuit travels down the right leg from the lower dantian and passes through the Earth to return via the left foot.

1 *Sit on a chair and visualize the sun setting over a lake, tinting it gold. The lake is at the level of your lower dantian, and it spills over, pouring golden liquid down your right thigh, through your knee, and down the leg.*

2 *Visualize the liquid ebbing away through the yongquan gateway in your right foot— and disappear into the Earth. It moves underground before rising through the yongquan center in your left foot, and up the leg, back to the dantian, where it fills the lake. This visualization should last 3 minutes at first, building up to about 10 minutes.*

WHITE CRANE

This chapter illustrates a sequence of QiGong exercises, collectively called a form. The name of this *form* is White Crane, since many of the exercises imitate the movements of the crane—its one-legged stance when searching for food in its marshland habitat, the darting forward of its head when securing its prey, the undulations of its wings in flight. This version of White Crane is one of many styles of QiGong based on the imitation of birds and animals. Learning a form is a good way of beginning QiGong because it teaches you the patterns of movement and mental awareness which are its essence. If you set aside regular times to learn and practice the form you will quickly absorb the movements, body and mind, so they become second nature.

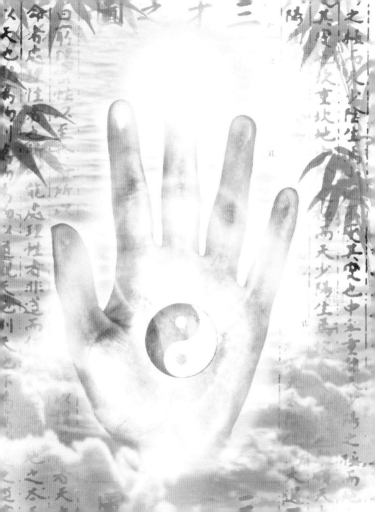

Introducing the Form

A form is a sequence of preset movements, which you learn and practice in a given order. The exercises follow a pattern so they are easy to learn, and because the movements are choreographed, a form has a finite length. This form has 128 movements, divided into five sets or parts. In the following pages the movements in each part are broken down into separate exercises short enough to learn in one practice session of perhaps half an hour. The color pages explain each exercise step by step, and the details of the exercises on the color pages are analyzed on the black and white pages that follow. With regular practice it should take about three months to learn the whole form, and when you have mastered it, the entire movement sequence takes 30–40 minutes to perform.

There are several versions of White Crane, and the one presented in these pages is especially good for beginners because the movements are varied and well balanced.

Practice time

Thirty to forty minutes is a good length for a form because it gives time for awareness to focus, emerge, develop, and ripen. However, although it is best to practice QiGong every day, you may not want or have time to go through the whole form. It is enough to repeat a few exercises or a standing meditation for a few minutes daily to keep the breathing, the body, and the mind honed and loosened. That alone will relax you and improve your concentration. But continuity is essential, so when you have learned the whole form, be sure to run through it at least once a week.

Awareness and visualization

The form exercises the whole body, directing awareness from hands to head to feet. In QiGong, awareness of energy flow is as important as physical movement, so each exercise is not only analyzed but guidelines are given for the visualizations that accompany them. Many visualizations are illustrated to help readers who are new to this way of exercising.

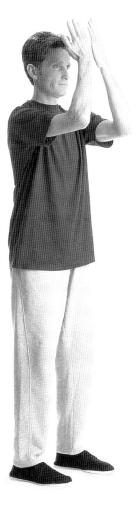

Third Eye

The Third Eye is a short movement sequence that may be practiced independently of the form. Movement sequences are broken down into steps in the following pages only to make it easy to learn the exercise. When you practice, your hands and arms should rise from your hips to head and back in one flowing movement.

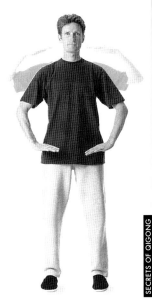

WHITE CRANE PART 1

The form begins with a standing meditation before stretching and exercising the upper body and deepening the breathing. The arm undulations on the first pages are tiny, fluid movements. Work at achieving them but bear in mind that the key to fine movement in QiGong is to remain relaxed and flexible, and to make the effort to visualize the movement rather than rely on mere physical effort to achieve it. In Push Back and Throw, which follows, you release pent-up energy in a vigorous motion. The arm movements are larger here, but maintain control. Energy must be released smoothly, and this throw depends on good coordination of all parts of the body. Maintain the coordination and flow as you lift your hands to press Qi into the crown energy center, and when pressing to Earth. In these final exercises you stretch up and bend, twist and turn before coming to rest in a standing meditation at the end.

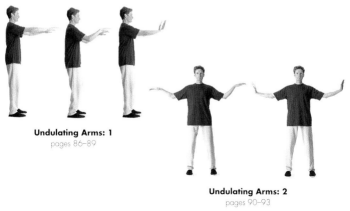

Undulating Arms: 1
pages 86–89

Undulating Arms: 2
pages 90–93

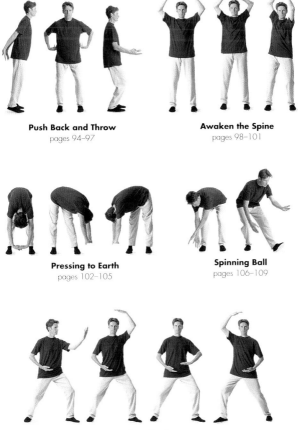

Push Back and Throw
pages 94–97

Awaken the Spine
pages 98–101

Pressing to Earth
pages 102–105

Spinning Ball
pages 106–109

Drawing In
pages 110–113

A Standing Meditation

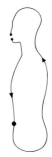

Each part of the form begins and ends with a simple standing posture, a standing meditation lasting for a minute or more. These are important moments in the form, because they provide a transition between the outer world of your everyday life and the inner world of QiGong.

Standing for a minute before you begin the first exercise enables you to focus on breathing and to develop a sense of the microcosmic orbit. Your movements will flow only if your body is relaxed, so take a moment to lift your shoulders and drop them into their natural position, to stretch up, relaxing your back, to lift your head and look forward, keeping your eyes open and relaxed, focusing on the middle distance.

Visualizing energy

The purpose of QiGong is to cultivate the flow of energy around the body. During the standing meditation you need to focus your mind on the pathway the Qi will be taking when you begin the exercises. Direct your mind to the lower

The Microcosmic Orbit
Spend the first moments of Part 1 in standing meditation, feet hip-width apart, imagining the microcosmic orbit: your internal Qi rising from the lower dantian up your spine to the crown of your head, and down your face and the front of your body. Follow three or four turns of this wheel of life in your mind.

dantian, where the microcosmic orbit begins, and breathe into it. Concentrate your mind on feeling the energy travel along its pathway; the movements you are about to begin will work on enhancing that circulation and increasing your body's internal energy store. Think of the limits of your body and imagine the Qi emanating beyond your corporeal self to form an aura around you, an interface between the inner circuit of Qi and the greater Qi from the external world surrounding you.

When the palms are open, the laogong energy gateways in the center draw external energy into the body

Branching Qi

When you have a strong sense of Qi following the microcosmic orbit, focus on the Qi branching as it reaches the top of the spine and traveling across the shoulders and down the arms to the laogong points in the palms of the hands.

UNDULATING ARMS: 1

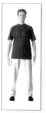

The form begins with small movements to stimulate the circulation of chi. Start in the basic standing posture shown on the left, with your feet shoulder-width apart and your arms by your sides, palms facing your thighs. The first steps introduce subtle, graceful arm movements whose rhythmic motion activates the communications circuit from the spinal cord to and from the limbs. The wavelike movements of elbows, wrists, and hands stretch the upper body from the spine out along the arms to the fingertips.

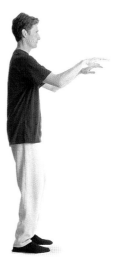

1 *From the basic standing posture shown top left, raise your arms in front of you to shoulder level, and turn the palms of your hands to face the ground, fingers and elbows straight but relaxed. Bending your knees, drop the base of your spine a fraction toward the floor.*

2 *Lifting your hands a fraction and keeping your arms relaxed, drop your elbows a little, bending them slightly to draw your arms toward your chest. As you do so, relax your hands from the wrist joints so that as they move toward you, they droop slightly.*

3 Now gently straighten your arms to push your hands away from your chest again, and as you do so, slowly straighten your legs so you rise a fraction, and open your palms.

Repeat and move on

Repeat steps 2 and 3 twice, then drop your hands to return to step 1, ready to make the first movement on page 90.

Elbows akimbo

Do not let your elbows stick out sideways as shown below. Keep them relaxed, pointing toward the ground, and press elbows and forearms gently inward, toward each other.

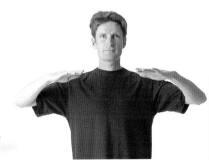

Beginning

A s you raise your arms in step 1 on page 86, focus your mind's eye on the lower dantian (see page 31) and visualize the intensity of your awareness boosting the circulation of Qi. The lower dantian is the point from which Qi rises up the spine. As your arms begin to draw in and out in steps 2 and 3, see it branch across your shoulders as you did in the standing meditation, and flow along your arms to your palms.

Stimulating energy flow

The rhythmic moving of your hands and arms and the rise and fall of your spine are the pump that stimulates this energy circuit. Relaxation rather than effort is the key to their gentle undulations. Do not pull your hands toward you in step 2 on page 86, so much as relax your shoulders and elbows, creating a downward movement that bends your arms slightly and pulls your hands toward you. And in step 3, rather than push your arms out, gently straighten your elbows and, while imperceptibly lifting your spine, let your palms open

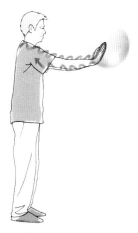

Rhythm of the waves

Qi ripples like wavelets from your shoulders, along your arms to your fingers, and washes back to your shoulders in a gentle rhythm. Shoulders ... hands ... shoulders ... hands ... a wave of energy bathing your arms.

out. The gentle flowing movement feels like liquid Qi rippling from your shoulders to your fingertips and back. After three undulations, pause with your arms stretched out in front, your hands, palms down, aligned with your wrists.

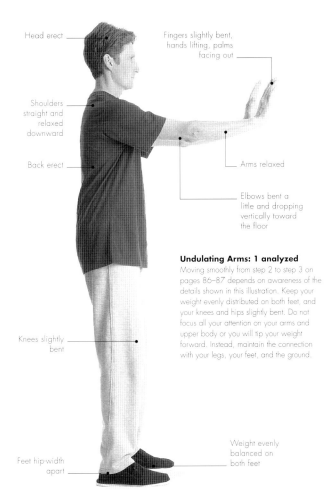

Head erect

Fingers slightly bent, hands lifting, palms facing out

Shoulders straight and relaxed downward

Back erect

Arms relaxed

Elbows bent a little and dropping vertically toward the floor

Undulating Arms: 1 analyzed

Moving smoothly from step 2 to step 3 on pages 86–87 depends on awareness of the details shown in this illustration. Keep your weight evenly distributed on both feet, and your knees and hips slightly bent. Do not focus all your attention on your arms and upper body or you will tip your weight forward. Instead, maintain the connection with your legs, your feet, and the ground.

Knees slightly bent

Weight evenly balanced on both feet

Feet hip-width apart

UNDULATING ARMS: 2

The form continues the wavelike arm movements shown on pages 86–87, but this time your arms stretch out to the sides. The undulations increase the flow of Qi up the spine and along the arms from the shoulders to the hands and back, opening the meridians in the shoulders and the arms. It also exercises the joints of the shoulders, the elbows, and the wrists without straining them, and it flexes and extends the many joints of the hands.

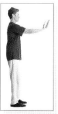

Start position

Start from your position at the end of the last movement sequence: step 3 on page 87.

1 *Keeping your hands, palms down, aligned with your wrists, open both arms out in an arc, imagining your fingertips feeling around the horizon, until your arms are stretched out to the sides. Relax your shoulders and elbows.*

3 Now gently straighten your arms to push your hands away from your shoulders again, and as you do so, slowly straighten your legs so you rise a fraction, and lift your hands to open your palms until they face outward.

Repeat and move on
Repeat steps 2 and 3 twice, making smooth undulations with your arms, then drop your hands to return to step 1.

2 Lift both hands until the palms face out. Keeping your elbows relaxed, bend them a little, and drop them slightly to draw your arms toward your shoulders. Drop your seat by a fraction toward the floor. As your hands move toward your shoulders let them droop from the wrists.

Making Waves

From making wavelike movements with your arms stretched out in front on pages 86–87, open with scarcely a pause into the rhythmic sideways movements on pages 90–91. You may need to practice the seamless transition from arms out in front to arms opened out to the sides. Follow the pathway of the Qi in your mind's eye, straightening your legs a little and lifting your seat slightly as the Qi rises up your spine like liquid rising up the scale of a thermometer. As your arms begin to move, imagine the Qi as a liquid washing back and forth from your shoulders to your hands. See the crest of a wave rolling out to your fingertips as you push out, and the undertow pulling your hands back toward your body.

Energizing actions

The rhythmic motion of your arms activates the body's communications circuit from the spinal cord and its major branching nerves to and from the limbs. Their gentle movements make your whole body feel energized, full of

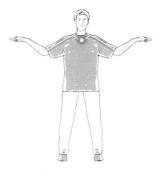

Illuminating energy

In step 3 you push outwards, as if against two shadows pressing in on either side. Visualize the waves of Qi rippling out from your spine along each arm and a light turning on in each palm as the Qi reaches it.

lifegiving Qi. Stretching the arms out opens the upper spine—the lightning rod for the body's energy—releasing the Qi along the meridian pathways to the upper limbs. As you repeat the movement for the third time, your arms, elbows, wrists, palms, and fingers will seem almost to have a life of their own and as you finish will move effortlessly back to their position at the end of step 1.

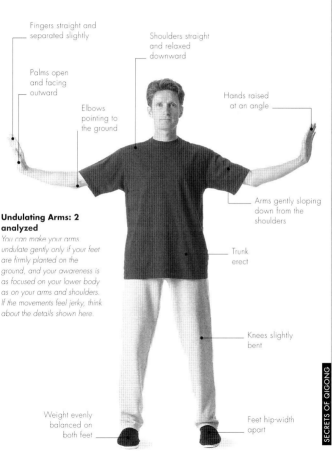

Fingers straight and
separated slightly

Shoulders straight
and relaxed
downward

Palms open
and facing
outward

Hands raised
at an angle

Elbows
pointing to
the ground

Arms gently sloping
down from the
shoulders

**Undulating Arms: 2
analyzed**

*You can make your arms
undulate gently only if your feet
are firmly planted on the
ground, and your awareness is
as focused on your lower body
as on your arms and shoulders.
If the movements feel jerky, think
about the details shown here.*

Trunk
erect

Knees slightly
bent

Weight evenly
balanced on
both feet

Feet hip-width
apart

PUSH BACK AND THROW

This dynamic exercise appears when the whole body has been energized. Its purpose is to clear stale Qi from the body and eject it into the world beyond. This is the first of two appearances in the form of Push Back and Throw. Here its cleansing role prepares the body for movement sequences that stimulate breathing and are said to be able to relieve heart disease and lung disorders, such as emphysema.

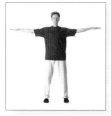

Start position
You start from your position at the end of step 1 on page 90.

1 *Keeping your shoulders and arms straight but relaxed, lower your arms level with your thighs and rotate your hands so the palms face back.*

2 *Lifting your heels slightly, push your whole body forward from your ankles, as if pushing against a wall of air, and extend your arms and hands back behind you.*

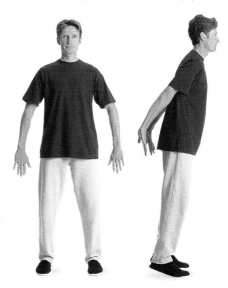

3 Keeping your body leaning forward and heels lifted, bend your knees slightly, bend your elbows out to the sides, and, little fingers leading, lift your hands as high as you can toward your armpits.

4 Now turn your hands outward, your palms up, while thrusting your hands forward as if shaking something off your palms. Drop your heels to the ground with a gentle bump, to stand upright again. Your hands come to rest, palms still facing up, roughly at hip level.

As you propel your hands forward from your armpits in step 3, move your thumbs across the palms to touch the base of the fourth or little fingers. This is a containing action intended to stop the release of Qi from the laogong points.

95

Clearing Stale Qi

The energizing effect of the arm movements in the foregoing exercises produces a feeling of completeness as you bring your hands down beside your thighs, ready to push back and throw on page 94. In step 2 you incline your body forward while keeping your heels lifted, weight on the forefeet, as if leaning into a high wind whose force keeps you upright. You push your arms and hands back into the space behind your kidneys.

Eliminating stale Qi

The kidneys are associated with the elimination of wastes from the body, so as you raise your hands in step 3, visualize them lifting and drawing out stale Qi trapped in your body systems and releasing it with an energetic throw beyond the body's outer limits. Imagine the movements of your arms behind your back as a gathering of negative forces, and the throw as a clearing-out of used or negative Qi. The action of placing the thumbs at the base of the fourth fingers ensures that positive

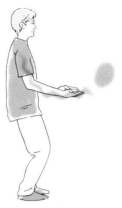

Clearing the system
As you prepare to throw, imagine yourself casting fatigue from your mind or expelling pollutants from your tissues, freeing pent-up emotions from your spirit, or releasing energy trapped in your meridians. Experience a release of tension as you jettison them outward.

Qi does not escape. Experience this exercise as a release of tension. Its result will be to spread the energizing effect of the arm movements that precede it throughout your whole body. And it makes a connection between the Qi in your body and the external Qi.

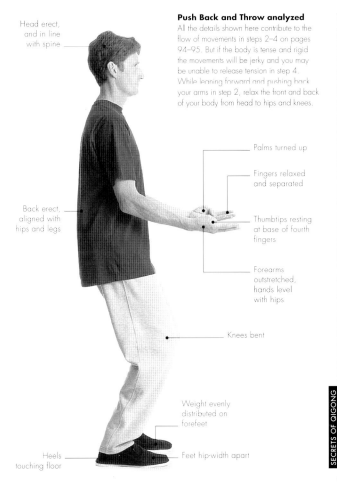

Head erect, and in line with spine

Push Back and Throw analyzed

All the details shown here contribute to the flow of movements in steps 2–4 on pages 94–95. But if the body is tense and rigid the movements will be jerky and you may be unable to release tension in step 4. While leaning forward and pushing back your arms in step 2, relax the front and back of your body from head to hips and knees.

Palms turned up

Fingers relaxed and separated

Thumbtips resting at base of fourth fingers

Back erect, aligned with hips and legs

Forearms outstretched, hands level with hips

Knees bent

Weight evenly distributed on forefeet

Heels touching floor

Feet hip-width apart

AWAKEN THE SPINE

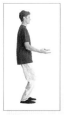

It is the turn of the upper spine and the shoulders to be exercised in these movements. First, energy is gathered and raised to the head, from where it dissolves into the body through the crown energy center. The movements that follow stretch the shoulder girdle in all directions, rotating the neck and the shoulders. Mental fatigue, depression, insomnia, and Chronic Fatigue Syntrome may all respond to this stimulation of the upper body combined with focused awareness on each part of the spine in turn.

Start position
You finished the throw on page 95 standing with your hands held out hip level, palms facing up.

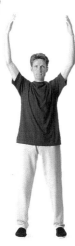

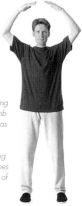

1 Raise your hands until they are high above your head, straightening your arms and releasing your thumb from the base of your little fingers as you lift.

2 Cup your hands a little and bring them forwards to rest about 6 inches (15 centimeters) above the crown of your head.

4 Bending your knees a little, drop your spine 2 inches (5 centimeters) and with your fingers still interlocked, palms facing up, stretch your hands about 9 inches (20 centimeters) above your crown. First moving your left shoulder forward and the right shoulder back, repeat the paddling movement in step 3.

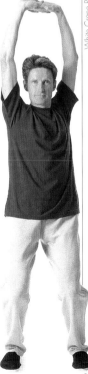

5 Bend your knees a little more, drop your spine 4 inches (10 centimeters) and stretch your interlocked hands about 12 inches (30 centimeters) above your crown. Start by moving your right shoulder forward and your left shoulder back, and paddle your elbows three times.

Repeat and move on
Now bring both elbows back in line with your ears, and sitting deeply into the stance but without dropping your seat further, stretch up once from your tail to your fingers.

3 Join your hands, interlocking the fingers, and turn the palms to face up. Move your right shoulder forward and your left shoulder back, then your left shoulder forward and your right shoulder back, and then move your right shoulder forward again, and your left shoulder back.

Replenishing Energy

As you rest in the neutral position after the throw on page 95, your thumbs still touch the base of the fourth finger of each hand, so containing the good Qi remaining inside the body. Releasing your thumbs enables you to lift fresh energizing Qi to the top of your head. Bring your hands closer to your crown center and let the Qi pour through it and dissolve back into your body. The Qi circulates first to your shoulders which, filled with energy, feel loose and flowing, ready to lead the paddling movements which follow.

Rotating the spine

If you keep your eyes fixed on a point straight in front, the paddling of your shoulders and arms in step 2 rotates your neck. Focus your mind on your neck; and as you paddle your arms in step 3, focus on your shoulders. This time, you rotate the thoracic vertebrae of the upper to mid-spine. Then, as you lower your hips still further in step 4, and raise your hands to their highest point, direct your awareness to your

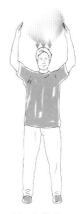

A golden ball of energy
Visualize yourself in steps 1 and 2 on page 98 lifting a shining golden ball of energy and bringing it to rest above your head. Imagine the warm energy flowing into the crown energy centers and melting down through your body.

lower back. The paddling of your shoulders and arms exercises the spine from your lower back to the sacrum at the base. Concentrate on dropping the spine and bending the legs just a fraction more each time to increase the intensity of the stretch.

Fingers interlocked, palms turned up

Hands about 6 inches (15 centimeters) above crown of head

Head upright, in line with spine

Eyes unmoving, focused on a fixed point straight ahead

Arms paddling, right elbow moving first

Shoulders leading arm movements

Awaken the Spine analyzed

Achieving gentle, fluid movements when you paddle your arms in steps 3–5 of Awaken the Spine on pages 98–99 depends on a solid sense of alignment that descends from your hands, through the crown of your head to your sacrum. Your feet need to be firmly planted, your buttocks tucked in, and your sitting bones stretching down toward the floor. Hold your head lightly and relax all parts of your body down to your toes.

Knees bent

Feet hip-width apart, firmly planted

Weight evenly balanced on both feet

PRESSING TO EARTH

In this exercise you bend down to press accumulated energy into the ground, connecting with the Earth through your hands as well as your feet. A physical effect of this movement is to stretch your lower back and the muscles at the backs of your thighs, which may well have become stiff through lack of exercise and poor posture. As well as eliminating back pain, these movements are said by some authorities to relieve digestive problems and, because bending and rising massages the colon, disorders of the intestines.

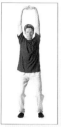

Start position
Begin with your knees bent, back and head erect, arms straight, hands stretching above your head, fingers interlocked, and palms turned upward.

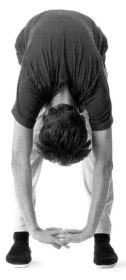

1 *Relax your elbows, straighten your legs, and bend forward from the hips. Tuck your head between your shoulders to align it with your spine and stretch down toward the ground as far as you comfortably can without straining.*

2 Bend your knees, raise your back a little, and turn to the left. Keeping your joined hands pressing downward from the crown of your head, press your palms down toward the ground.

3 Again, bend your legs and lift from the hips to raise your back a little, and this time swivel to the right before pressing your interlocked fingers down to the ground for a third time.

Finish and move on
Bend your knees to raise your back and turn to the front, then instead of pressing downward again, rise into a crouching position.

Earth Connection

When performing the movements on pages 102–103 it is as if you are directing the Qi which you poured into your body through the crown center on pages 98–99 down into the ground, and pressing the Earth around the spot where you planted it. Imagine that, in later exercises, you may reap a harvest of fresh Qi energy from that same spot.

Stretching the hamstrings

Bending forward while pressing your interlocked fingers, palms turned out, toward the ground on pages 102–103 stretches the hamstrings—three muscles at the backs of the thighs with long, tough tendons. These tendons tighten if they are not stretched regularly, and bending forward will help to loosen them. If you have to stand for long periods at work, these movements will help relieve backache. They are also especially necessary for anyone who has to sit for prolonged periods at work. However, if you rarely bend or exercise your spine, take care at first. Bend

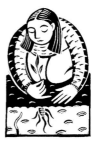

Planting Qi

The intensity of your stretch shows in your hands pressing to Earth. Imagine yourself bending to firm the soil around a seedling of Qi you have just planted.

forward from the hips, keeping your back straight. If you bend from your waist you put strain on your upper back. You may strain your lower back if you try to push your hands to the floor, so bend only as far as is comfortable—if your back is very supple your hands should reach the level of your ankles. If your back feels stiff, practicing this exercise every other day will improve its elasticity. Finally, always bend your legs before lifting your back from a forward bend to avoid straining the lumbar vertebrae.

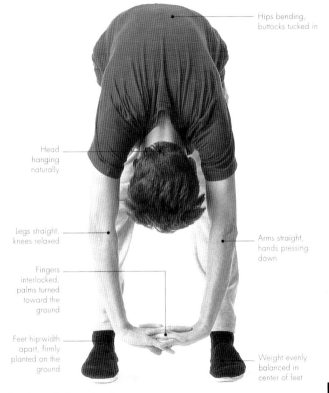

Hips bending,
buttocks tucked in

Head
hanging
naturally

Legs straight,
knees relaxed

Arms straight,
hands pressing
down

Fingers
interlocked,
palms turned
toward the
ground

Feet hip-width
apart, firmly
planted on the
ground

Weight evenly
balanced in
center of feet

Pressing to Earth analyzed

Check each point in this illustration before practicing
the movements on pages 102–103, then check each
one again in your mind as you bend forward in steps
1–3. If possible, ask a teacher, a friend, or even look
in a mirror to see that your upper back is as straight as
possible and that you are not bending from the waist.

SPINNING BALL

As you complete the last movements of Pressing to Earth on page 103, a ball of energy begins to appear between your hands. Now you spin the ball, directing your attention outward as you move your body from right to left, twisting and rotating your spine. This exercise completes the sequence of movements that works on loosening the spine at the core of the body, opening it up to other complex movements later in the form.

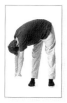

Start position
Start with your feet hip-width apart, legs bent into a crouch, trunk bending to the right, hands interlocked, palms pressing down.

1 *Unclasp your hands and move your left hand 12 inches (30 centimeters) in front of your right hand. Leading with the fourth finger of your left hand and right first finger, gather the ball of energy and start to spin it to the left, bending your right leg.*

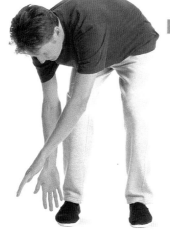

Direction-finding

Imagine a compass inscribed on the floor of the room in which you stand, and start each sequence of movements facing north. As you spin the ball, turn to the northwest diagonal and step along it with your left foot.

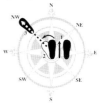

2 As you begin to spin the ball you transfer 60 percent of your weight to your right leg. Now lift your left heel and turn slowly to the left, pivoting on the ball of your left foot and moving the spinning ball leftward.

3 As your left foot pivots to point northwest, the ball grows, pushing your palms about 18 inches (45 centimeters) apart. As you complete the turn, begin to straighten your legs and step with your left foot along the northwest diagonal. Your right arm starts to rise as your heel touches the ground.

Moving Qi

Be ready as you unclasp your interlocked fingers in step 1 on page106 to visualize a golden ball of energy to appear between them. In Pressing to Earth on page 103, the palms of your clasped hands were facing the ground and connecting with the Earth, so perhaps they pulled the ball of Earth energy with them as they rose. The ball grows in your hands, which move apart to hold it, the left hand moving out to the front before circling to the back, and the right hand circling to the front, finishing with the palms facing each other. You transfer your weight to your bent right leg as the ball expands. It touches the ground, and with your hands you set it spinning.

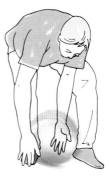

Rotating energy

Your moving hands set the globe of golden energy spinning on the ground, and orbiting like the Earth along an arc stretching from the north to the northwest.

Orbiting Qi

Crouching on your right leg and lifting your left heel, you send the spinning ball in an arc to the left, rotating on the ball of your left foot to follow its orbit with your upper body. As you finish, your left foot and knee and your upper body all face the northwest diagonal.

Watch the ball and direct your mind toward it as you spin it. Pivot at a measured pace, keeping a sense of rhythm, turning your hands as you rotate your body. As you complete the movement your left foot steps along the northwest diagonal and your left hand comes to rest in front of your left ankle, palm facing north, with your right hand ahead of it, palms facing each other.

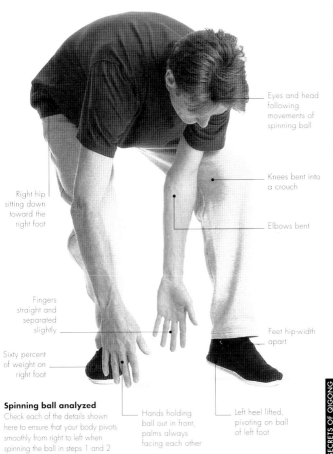

Eyes and head
following
movements of
spinning ball

Knees bent into
a crouch

Elbows bent

Right hip
sitting down
toward the
right foot

Feet hip-width
apart

Fingers
straight and
separated
slightly

Sixty percent
of weight on
right foot

Spinning ball analyzed
Check each of the details shown
here to ensure that your body pivots
smoothly from right to left when
spinning the ball in steps 1 and 2
on pages 106–107.

Hands holding
ball out in front,
palms always
facing each other

Left heel lifted,
pivoting on ball
of left foot

DRAWING IN

You end the first part of the form by lifting the spinning ball of energy you created on pages 106–107 to your head to let it pour into the crown energy center, and down through your body to replenish your stores of internal Qi. You perform this movement twice, first on the left side, then on the right, before gathering your hands in toward the lower dantian and resting in the standing posture, palms turning up.

Start position

You face northwest with your weight on your right foot, left heel touching the floor ahead of it. Your right hand rests midway between your calves and your left hand is rising.

1 *Lower your left forefoot to the floor, toes pointing along the northwest diagonal. Scoop your right hand around to the right and rest it at the side, palm up. As your left hand reaches eye level, lift your head to look at the palm.*

2 *Transfer your gaze from your left palm toward the north and continue lifting your left hand until it rests palm down just above the crown of your head.*

4 *Transfer 60 percent of your weight to your left side and step with your right foot, placing it heel first on the northeast diagonal while raising your right hand to eye level and looking at the palm. Your left hand remains opposite the lower dantian.*

3 *Now lower your left hand slowly down the front of your body, palm facing down. When it reaches the level of the dantian, turn the palm up and rest it about 4 inches (10 centimeters) from your body.*

5 *Now look to the north and lift your right hand until it rests palm down over the crown of your head. Then drop your hand slowly down the right side of your body to rest it about 4 inches (10 centimeters) away from you opposite the lower dantian.*

Finish

When you raise your left hand at the beginning of the movement sequence on page 110, you lift the spinning globe of Qi lightly through the air to eye level, where you pause to look at it, concentrating on bringing the Qi to the palm of your left hand. Then, raising it higher, to the crown of your head, you release the liquid Qi into your crown center and let it pour slowly through your body, drawing it down to the lower dantian energy center. You carry out these movements twice, first facing the

Footwork

You finish step 3 with your left foot pointing northwest and your right foot a step behind it pointing north. In step 4 you take one step with your right foot along the northeast diagonal while pivoting your left foot until the toes point north. To finish part 1, simply step forward with your left foot, to align it with the right, and swivel your right foot to point north.

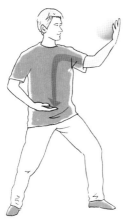

Showering Qi

As you lower your hand in steps 3 and 5, imagine warm Qi pouring down through the central energy channel of your body, and bathing your skin, warming you through.

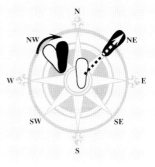

northwest diagonal, then stepping to the
northeast diagonal with your right foot,
and lifting the Qi with your right hand.

Each hand in turn guides the Qi
down the central energy channel to
the lower dantian and rests in front
of it ready to end Part 1 of the form.
You finish in the classic stance with
your hands in their natural resting
position, palms turned up opposite
the lower dantian, feet parallel, and
eyes directed ahead. Pause briefly,
calmly visualizing the Qi gathering in
your body and circulating around it.

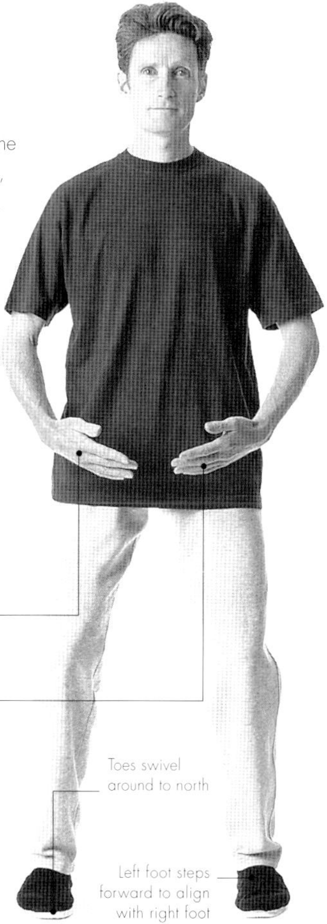

Right hand rests at level
of lower dantian, palm
turned up at 45° angle

Left hand comes to
rest at level of lower
mirroring right hand

Toes swivel
around to north

Final stance
End the sequence by stepping up to bring
the back (left) foot in line with your right foot,
and draw your hands to rest palms up close
to the abdomen. Straighten both legs, lift
from the base of your spine to the crown of
your head, and look straight ahead.

Left foot steps
forward to align
with right foot

WHITE CRANE PART 2

The theme of working the upper body continues in Part 2, but here the movements involve the hands as well as the arms. At the start of Magic Wand the fingers point forward in a powerful posture designed to direct energy outward. In the open hand exercises that follow, the palms come into play and need to be a focus of your awareness. In Holding Qi your palms turn to the sky to absorb new Qi; in the Third Eye they seem to lock onto the brow energy center as they press Qi into it; and in Gathering they touch down on the lung point near the shoulder joint, where they touch the lung meridian and so stimulate breathing.

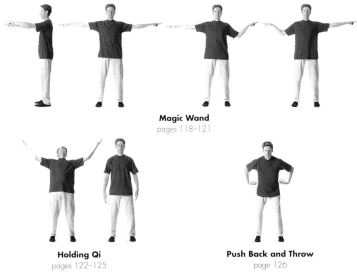

Magic Wand
pages 118–121

Holding Qi
pages 122–125

Push Back and Throw
page 126

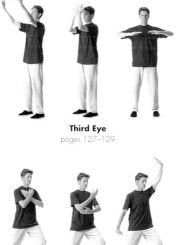

Third Eye
pages 127–129

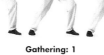

Gathering: 1
pages 130–133

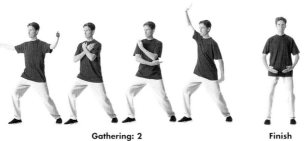

Gathering: 2
pages 134–137

Finish
pages 136–137

Opening the Lungs

Stretching the arms up above the head and tipping the head back as in Holding Qi on pages 122–123 opens the airways. It clears the sinuses (the air spaces around the nose) and stretches the front of the neck so your mouth opens. You breathe in almost involuntarily, taking air all the way into your lungs. As you lower your arms you automatically breathe out deeply. Hyperventilation—shallow breathing using only the upper part of the lungs, an increasingly common reaction to stress—is impossible when you perform this exercise.

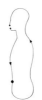

Microcosmic orbit
Begin Part 2 in a standing meditation visualizing the Qi pathway through your body. Here, it follows the microcosmic orbit, as in your preparation for Part 1 (see page 84).

Improved breathing

QiGong teaches you how to breathe well. Lifting, stretching up, and lowering the arms in Holding Qi and in the Third Eye, which follows it, stimulates your breathing. Gathering on pages 130–137 has the same effect from the inside. The action of cupping your hands and touching the lung point at the shoulder joint with the tip of the middle finger activates the lung meridian, and later in the same exercise you transfer fresh Qi into the meridian by laying the palm of each hand on the lung point.

The lungs suffer daily from poor air quality, pollution, and shallow breathing caused by stress and lack of aerobic exercise. Practising Part 2 of the form daily will help keep your lungs healthy and will improve your condition if you suffer from asthma, but rather than focus on your breathing, concentrate on moving smoothly and rhythmically and your breathing will adapt to the rhythm.

Lung meridian

The lung meridian
occurs on the right
and left of the body.
It begins on the upper
chest opposite the
armpit, travels around
the front of the shoulder,
down the outside of the
arm, and ends on the
thumbnail.

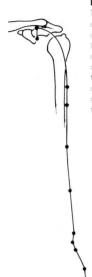

Laogong point

Standing meditation

*Spend a few moments visualizing internal Qi
circulating around the microcosmic orbit, then
imagine it branching at the top of your spine
across your shoulders and along your arms to finish
at the laogong point in the center of each palm.*

MAGIC WAND

Part 2 of the form begins with undulating arm movements that send internal Qi circulating across your shoulders and down into your arms and hands. Here, however, the movements are led not by open palms as they were in Part 1, but by two pointing fingers, a powerful hand shape for directing energy outward from the meridians. The movements are gentle and rhythmic, but they build strength in the muscles of the arms and shoulders just as much as weight-training might do, and they improve the flexibility of the shoulder area.

1 From the standing posture, knees slightly bent, palms facing thighs, raise both arms in front of you to shoulder level, elbows pointing down and pressing toward each other. Make the magic wand (see right) with your fingers, and rotate your wrists inward until the palms face down.

2 Keeping your arms raised to shoulder level and your hands in line with your wrists, slowly open your arms in an arc as if tracing the line of the horizon with your pointing fingers, until your arms and shoulders form a straight line from fingertip to fingertip.

3 Begin the arm movements by relaxing your left shoulder and dropping the left elbow slightly, pulling the hand in briefly.

4 Straighten your left elbow to push the hand outward, while relaxing your right shoulder and dropping the elbow slightly to pull your right hand in toward your shoulder.

5 Now straighten your right elbow to push the right hand out, while relaxing your left shoulder and dropping the left elbow to pull your left hand in again.

Making the magic wand

Curl down the third and fourth finger of each hand until the tips touch the palms, place the tip of each thumb on the joint of the third finger, and point the first two fingers forward.

Repeat and move on

Keeping your elbows relaxed, your arms at shoulder height, and your fingers pointing out to the sides, repeat step 4, then step 5, then step 4 again, making smooth, wavelike movements with your arms. Then straighten your right arm to return to your position in step 2.

Directing Energy

When you open your arms wide after creating the magic wand with your hands in the first movements on page 118, imagine your arms connected by a cord of Qi that stretches from fingertip to fingertip, along each arm and across your shoulders. As you move your arms and hands, the cord pulls the Qi from left hand to right hand, in much the same way as your fingers pull a bath towel across your back to dry it. Pulling your hands in and out pulls the Qi all the way across, back and forth, opening the meridians and energizing your arms by sending the Qi flowing down to each hand.

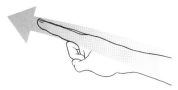

Using the magic wand
The name of this exercise is taken from the sword form in taijiquan (t'ai chi ch'uan), where pointing the fingers in the way shown here is used whenever the player intends to direct energy somewhere.

Energy rising

Be aware of being rooted like a tree to the Earth, and of Earth energy rising through your feet and up your legs to your spine, your main trunk. As you move your arms, feel it branch along them to reach the magic wand formed by your fingers, ready to be directed outward wherever you need to send it.

Moving your arms gently in and out as if they were riding out on the crest of a wave and pulling back with the undertow may seem more difficult when the palms of your hands are not lifting and falling as they were in Part 1. By now, however, you should find it more natural to relax your whole body before beginning the movements. Visualizing waves of Qi traveling along your arms to your hands and washing gently back gives you the feeling that leads the movement. It is as if you allow your arms and hands to move in and out rather than pull and push them.

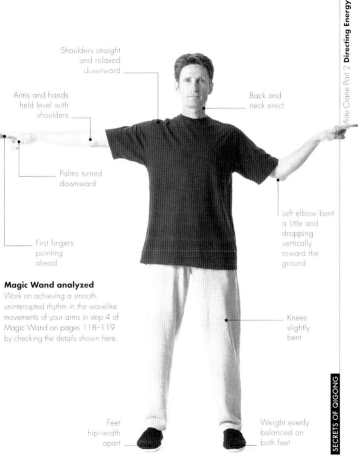

Shoulders straight
and relaxed
downward

Arms and hands
held level with
shoulders

Back and
neck erect

Palms turned
downward

First fingers
pointing
ahead

Left elbow bent
a little and
dropping
vertically
toward the
ground

Magic Wand analyzed

Work on achieving a smooth,
uninterrupted rhythm in the wavelike
movements of your arms in step 4 of
Magic Wand on pages 118–119
by checking the details shown here.

Knees
slightly
bent

Feet
hip–width
apart

Weight evenly
balanced on
both feet

HOLDING QI

Now you release your fingers from the magic wand formed on pages 118–119 and raise your outstretched arms to hold a huge ball of energy which tumbles from the sky. In the effort to hold it up you bend your spine right back, from the sacrum at the base to the atlas at the top. Bending the back stretches every vertebra, keeping your spine elastic. This exuberant, welcoming, accepting gesture opens the lungs and deepens the breathing, increasing the oxygen supply to the brain, and lifting depressed spirits.

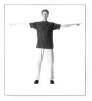

Start position
Begin standing with your feet parallel, your arms stretched out in line with your shoulders, your hands forming the magic wand.

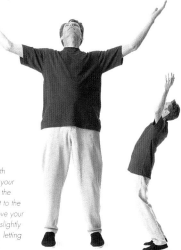

1 *Releasing your thumb and third and fourth fingers from the magic wand, but keeping your arms outstretched, rotate your wrists to turn the palms of your hands up, move your weight to the balls of your feet, and raise your arms above your head. Lift your heels and bend your knees slightly to incline your body back from the sacrum, letting your head fall back and your mouth open.*

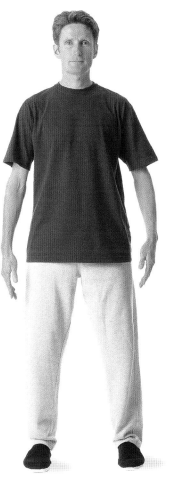

2 Lift your upper body, straighten your legs, and drop back on your heels to stand upright. At the same time, lower your arms to your sides, rotating your wrists to turn the palms to face down. Rest your hands a short distance from your thighs, palms facing your thighs.

Gathering the Cosmos

Open your arms to the sky in Holding Qi on pages 122–123, and they gather in cosmic Qi in the form of a ball. Holding the ball opens major energy centers—the third eye, the throat, and the heart.

Bending backward

To hold such a huge ball you must stretch your spine, your shoulders, and your head right back, and raise your arms and hands up and out to the sides. To achieve this, you must ground yourself firmly, so rather than concentrate on your arms and head, begin by focusing on your lower body. This is especially helpful for the many people who tend to resist bending backward. Check that your weight is evenly distributed on both feet, then move it forward, lifting your heels when you feel balanced. Bending your knees and lowering your pelvis makes you feel solidly grounded. Straighten your spine by stretching it from the sacrum to the atlas, open your arms wider, and move your shoulders back. When you feel confident, let your

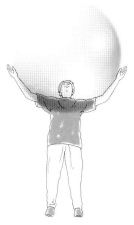

Capturing cosmic Qi
Visualize yourself spreading your arms wide to hold a huge ball of shining Qi up high. Imagine warm energy radiating down from the ball, warming your hands and head, and melting through your body.

head fall back and relax your neck and jaw, allowing your mouth to open. Feel the stretch up the front of your body to your chin. To finish, lower your arms to your sides to let the energy wash down your body, turning the palms down.

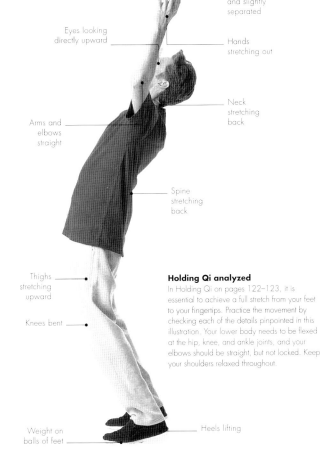

Fingers straight
and slightly
separated

Eyes looking
directly upward

Hands
stretching out

Neck
stretching
back

Arms and
elbows
straight

Spine
stretching
back

Thighs
stretching
upward

Knees bent

Holding Qi analyzed

In Holding Qi on pages 122–123, it is
essential to achieve a full stretch from your feet
to your fingertips. Practice the movement by
checking each of the details pinpointed in this
illustration. Your lower body needs to be flexed
at the hip, knee, and ankle joints, and your
elbows should be straight, but not locked. Keep
your shoulders relaxed throughout.

Weight on
balls of feet

Heels lifting

THE THIRD EYE

Lifting and holding Qi on pages 122–123 is immediately followed by a cleansing movement, the second appearance of Push Back and Throw, in which negative Qi is firmly expelled from the body. It is followed in its turn by a sequence of replenishing movements in which you raise Qi to the yin dang or brow center. This is often called the third eye because it resides in the center of the forehead between the eyebrows. The invigorating arm movements in these exercises relieve stress and awaken the senses.

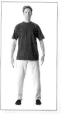

Start position
Begin with your feet hip-width apart, legs and arms straight, hands resting a few inches from your thighs.

Push Back and Throw
Turn your palms to face back, lift your heels, push your body forward extending your arms behind you, lift your hands toward your armpits; then thrust them forward in Push Back and Throw, shown on pages 94–95. Your hands finish roughly at hip level, palms facing up, thumbs touching the bases of the fourth fingers.

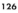

The Third Eye

1 *From the standing position at the end of the throw, straighten your legs and raise your hands to your head, extending your arms and releasing your thumbs from the bases of your fourth fingers as you lift up.*

third eye

2 *Bend your elbows to tip your hands toward your brow, so that hands and forehead form a triangle. Lift your head to look at your palms, then cup your hands a little, and move your elbows together to press the Qi into your brow center.*

3 *Complete the sequence by moving your elbows out to the sides a little, and moving your hands down level with your shoulders, rotating your wrists until the palms face down, then lower your hands toward the lower dantian.*

Awakening Vision

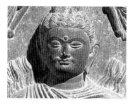

Stimulating vision
Imagine yourself pressing energy into a third eye projecting from the center of your brow, and that energy bathing, refreshing, and warming your eyes and your brain. Indigo is the color associated with this energy center.

Qi is the breath of life, and just as depleted air must be expelled from the lungs before fresh air can be introduced, so must the mind and body be cleared of spent, negative Qi before the fresh Qi gathered from the cosmos on pages 122–123 can be introduced to refresh and replenish. Begin the sequence of movements on pages 126–127 by concentrating hard on expelling all negative forces from within as you push back, gather used Qi, and cast it vigorously outward in Push Back and Throw. Follow the steps described and illustrated on pages 94–95 exactly, and work on moving without a break into step 1 of the Third Eye.

Replenishing Qi

Like punctuation in a sentence, this exercise recurs several times in the form. Here, its function is to replenish the body's store of internal Qi. Visualizing the action of lifting Qi gathered from the cosmos and sending it, via the third eye, circulating down the body's central pillar—the spine—should not be a difficult exercise because the yin dang or brow energy center is associated with vision and visualization, imagery and imagination. Pressing the elbows closer together in step 2 produces a spiraling movement of the palms which brings the Qi into contact with the third eye.

Complete the movements of this part of the form with your hands resting palms down opposite the lower dantian, the starting point for the circulation of internal Qi through the body.

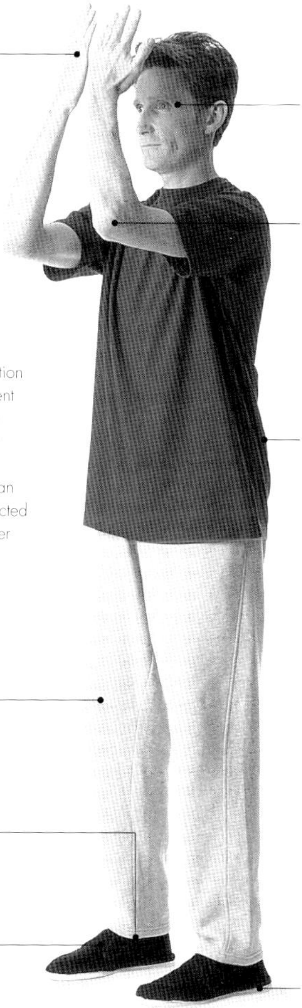

Hands about 6 inches (15 centimeters) from brow, fingers almost touching

Eyes looking at wrists

Elbows bent and moving in toward each other

Back straight, buttocks tucked in

Third Eye analyzed

Each of the points shown in this illustration contribute to the solid sense of alignment you need in step 2 of the Third Eye on page 127. Your feet need to be firmly planted and your knees and hip joints slightly flexed to ground you, so you can focus your attention on the energy directed by your hands through your brow center and down to the base of your spine.

Knees slightly bent

Feet hip-width apart, firmly planted

Weight evenly balanced on both feet

Heels firmly planted on ground

GATHERING: 1

Part 2 of the form ends with a sequence of movements that gather external Qi in from the cosmos and from the Earth. This exercise is performed first on the left side (as shown on these pages), turning toward the northwest diagonal; then on the right side, turning to the northeast diagonal (shown on pages 134–135). Stepping and turning to left and right, and raising one hand while pushing down with the other stimulates the spine, exercises the lungs, energizes the whole body, and improves physical and mental coordination.

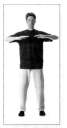

Start position
Begin standing with your feet hip-width apart, your hands moving, palms facing down, toward the lower dantian.

1 *Move your weight to your right leg, bend the knee, lift the left heel, and make a small turn to the northwest. Step forward with your left foot, placing the heel down first on the northwest diagonal and moving your weight forward as you do so. As your foot moves, swing both hands downward and arc them forward, turning the palms to face north.*

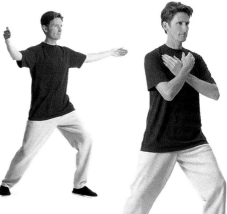

2 *Cupping both hands a little, swing your left hand in an arc across your chest and place the palm over the lung point at your right shoulder joint; then arc your right hand across your chest to place the palm over the left lung point.*

3 *Release your left hand and slide it down your chest beneath your right arm, around the right elbow. As your left hand clears your right elbow, begin lowering your right hand toward your right thigh.*

4 *Swing your left arm forward and up, turning the palm toward the diagonal as your fingers rise above your head. Bring your right hand to rest palm down beside your right thigh and in line with your right foot.*

Heaven to Earth

At the beginning of Gathering on page 130, the golden ball of Qi reappears between your hands as you swing your arms outward and turn the palms forward. Cupping each hand in turn, and swinging it across your chest, you energize your body by bringing fresh Qi to the lung points. Then, as your left hand is released from the lung point, it rounds the right elbow with a wiping motion, which clears spent Qi from inside the body and returns it to the external world.

Touching Heaven and Earth

The exercise reaches its conclusion in step 4, with a lifting of the left hand to the cosmos and a pressing of the right hand to the Earth. This vigorous stretch connects you to the Heaven above through your left palm and to the Earth beneath through your right palm, creating a simultaneous link which brings new external energy to be absorbed into the dantian.

This dynamic exercise in gathering does not end with this movement,

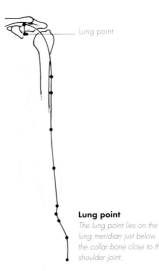

Lung point

Lung point
The lung point lies on the lung meridian just below the collar bone close to the shoulder joint.

however. Balance is a natural part of QiGong, so having completed the sequence of movements on the left, you then transfer your weight to the right side of your body and, as is shown on the following two pages, repeat the same movements on the right.

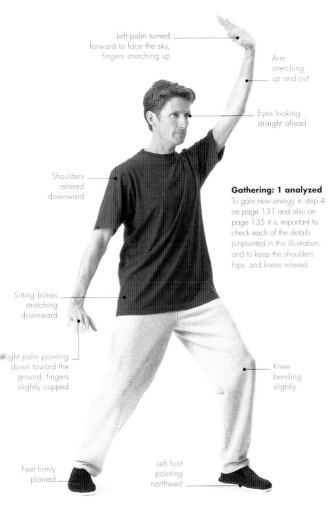

Left palm turned forward to face the sky, fingers stretching up

Arm stretching up and out

Eyes looking straight ahead

Shoulders relaxed downward

Gathering: 1 analyzed

To gain new energy in step 4 on page 131 and also on page 135 it is important to check each of the details pinpointed in this illustration, and to keep the shoulders, hips, and knees relaxed.

Sitting bones stretching downward

Right palm pointing down toward the ground, fingers slightly cupped

Knee bending slightly

Feet firmly planted

Left foot pointing northwest

GATHERING: 2

Here, the second part of the Gathering sequence which began on page 130 takes you in a different direction, for you perform the same movements on the right side of the body, stepping toward the northeast. Although you learn the sequence little by little, each step must melt seamlessly into the next, so that you move fluidly through the whole exercise from step 1 on page 130 to the final position on page 137.

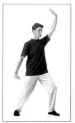

Start position
Your left hand is raised toward the northwest, your right palm faces the Earth, fingers pointing north. Your weight is on your left leg and your left toes point northwest.

1 *Turn your spine to the right and pivot on your left heel to point your left foot north. Moving all your weight to your left leg, step forward with your right foot, placing it heel first on the northeast diagonal, and move 60 percent of your weight forward. Meanwhile, raise your right hand, palm facing out, toward the northeast diagonal, and lower your left hand toward the northeast diagonal, palm facing out.*

2 *Closing your fingers a little to cup your hands, swing your right hand in an arc across your chest and place the palm over the lung point on your left shoulder; then arc your left hand across your chest to place the palm over the lung point on your right shoulder.*

3 Now release your right hand and slide it down your chest beneath your left arm, around the elbow. As your right hand clears your left elbow, begin moving your left hand down toward your left thigh.

4 Swing your right hand forward and up, turning the palm toward the diagonal as your hand rises above your head, and bring your left hand to rest palm down beside your thigh and facing north in line with your left foot.

Finish

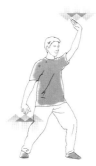

Making the connection

Connecting with Heaven and Earth simultaneously through the palms of the hands allows Qi to travel along the arms to the dantian energy center.

R ather than merely move your weight from your left leg to your right at the end of Gathering: 1 on page 131, move the balance of your body to the right side, so that when you pivot your foot, rotate your spine, and step to the northeast, you feel you have changed the direction of your mind as well as your body. You move your arms as you step, creating an open embrace toward the northeast.

The second phase of the exercise is a mirror image of the first, as you change the direction and repeat the movements, but on the opposite side of the body.

As you stretch one hand skyward and the other to the Earth to gather Qi, simply relax into yourself. Feel yourself

Footwork

You begin Gathering: 1 on page 131 facing north. Then, after turning your upper body toward the northwest in step 1, you lift your left foot and step along the northwest diagonal. At the start of Gathering: 2, pivot on the heel of your left foot to turn it to face north again, turn your spine toward the northeast, and step with your right foot along the northeast diagonal.

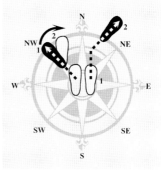

align with Heaven and Earth, connecting with them and conducting their energies through your body. As you complete Gathering: 2, however, draw your mind inward once again as you bring your hands to your sides and realign your feet, for you finish Part 2 of the form in the classic standing position, toes and heels aligned, eyes directed into the middle distance, hands resting, palms up, at the lower dantian, contemplating the external Qi you have just gathered circulating up through your body from the dantian energy center.

Right hand moves in toward lower dantian, palm turns up

Left hand moves in toward lower dantian, palm turns up

Completing Part 2

End the sequence by stepping forward with the (back) left foot and aligning both feet, heel to toe, facing north, and draw your hands to rest at the lower dantian, palms turned up at a 45° angle. Straighten both legs, lift from the base of your spine to the crown of your head, and look ahead.

Right foot steps forward to point north

Left foot pivots to align with right foot

WHITE CRANE PART 3

The focus of the form changes from the arms to the spine, beginning with wavelike motions of the head and neck, which imitate a crane searching out food. The lower body has a hidden but active role in the first exercises—bending the knees while craning the neck left and right pulls the spine from below, separating the lumbar vertebrae. The spinal stretch works the lower body still harder, extending the backs of the thighs while exercising the neck and head. Several exercises in this part of the form are performed with the hips and legs bent into a squat. This may be hard work at first, but your legs become much stronger as a result. Hip circles and knee rotations are weight-bearing exercises that help prevent bone loss and keep hips and knees flexible. If these joints are painful sit only as low as is comfortable. If you suffer from low back pain, focus on your alignment and on stretching up from the base of the spine.

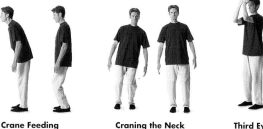

Crane Feeding
pages 142–145

Craning the Neck
pages 143–145

Third Eye
page 146

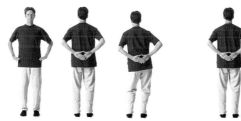

Hip Circles
page 147

Massaging the back
pages 148–149

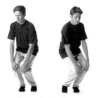

Knee Rotations
pages 150–153

Scissors
page 151

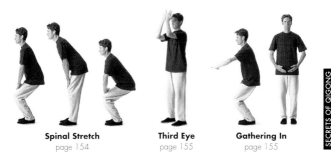

Spinal Stretch
page 154

Third Eye
page 155

Gathering In
page 155

White Circle **Part 3**

SECRETS OF QIGONG

139

Healing

All QiGong exercises help you stay fit and healthy, but Part 3 makes self-healing its special theme. Each of the exercises in the following 12 pages has a special power to strengthen weakness and remedy disorder in a particular area of the body and may be practiced outside the form as a solo exercise. For example, knee rotations on pages 154–157 when practiced as part of the form help prevent joint problems by working on the flexibility of the knees. If, however, you have stiff knees or if you are recovering from an injury, practice the rotations every day to restore the joint to health. Keeping the joints moving is an excellent antidote to degenerative disorders of the hips and knees, such as rheumatism and arthritis.

Crane Feeding which begins Part 3 massages and stimulates the thyroid, a gland which lies like a bowtie across the front of the neck and plays an important role in regulating metabolism, the body's utilization of energy from the food we eat.

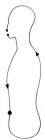

Qi pathway
Spend a minute at the beginning of Part 3 focusing on the pathway of the Qi. Instead of branching across the shoulders as in Parts 1 and 2, the Qi travels up the spine to the top of the head and down the front of the head and the body, linking the two central meridians. It finishes just below the lower lip at the top of the jen-mo meridian, but imagine a continuous circuit providing a pathway for the Qi to orbit the body.

Working on the spine

Almost all the exercises in this part of
the form, from Craning the Neck on
page 143 to Spinal Stretch on page
155, work on the spine, extending it
to counter the compressing effects of
gravity, and flexing and rotating the
many small muscles of the lower back.
Page 149 introduces the healing art
of self-massage, a branch of QiGong
called anmogong. Techniques for
massaging other parts of the body as
a form of self-healing are described
and illustrated in Chapter 5.

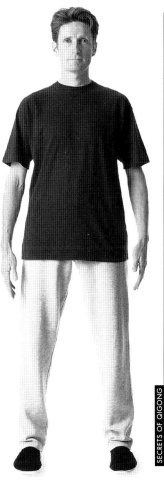

Standing meditation

Begin each part of the form in the basic standing
posture shown on page 37, relaxed but alert.
Keep your eyes open while visualizing the
pathway of the Qi shown opposite and in your
mind's eye watch for signs of the Qi circulating
around the body.

CRANE FEEDING

Part 3 of White Crane begins with a set of movements that imitate a crane feeding. It involves making small head movements, but it is also a holistic exercise that stretches the spine from bottom to top, countering the compressing effects of gravity, and exercises the muscles of the lower legs and the feet. It also massages the thyroid gland, which sits like a bowtie across the front of the windpipe in the neck and secretes a hormone that controls the body's production and use of energy.

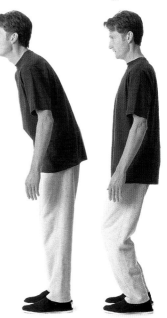

Crane Feeding

1 *Still standing as in the standing meditation on page 141, your feet a little less than hip-width apart and your hands by your sides, project your chin forward, then drop it toward your breastbone. Relax your jaw and let your mouth open.*

2 *Arch your chin back and tuck it in. Then, keeping your knees slightly bent, pull your head erect, as in step 1. Bend your legs and lower your pelvis a little further, then repeat steps 1 and 2, moving your head forward, down, back, and up. Then lower your pelvis still closer to the floor, as if sitting on an invisible chair, and repeat the same movements, smoothly drawing a circle in the air with your chin. Do not straighten your legs or raise your pelvis when lifting your head at the end.*

Craning the neck

Here, imitating the side-to-side movements a crane makes when stretching its neck up after feeding helps you rise from the low crouch at the end of Crane Feeding to a standing position.

1 *Lift the right side of your neck lightly up as if your head were being pulled up from the right temple, while straightening your legs and lifting your pelvis a fraction.*

2 *Stretch the left side of your neck up once more, while straightening your legs and lifting your pelvis a little more.*

Repeat and finish

Repeat steps 1 and 2 three times, straightening your legs a little further and lifting your pelvis a fraction more each time, so that after the sixth neck-stretch you are standing erect.

Head Movements

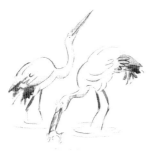

Imitating nature
Imagine yourself making the movements a crane makes when catching and swallowing its prey, and lifting its head to watch warily for danger.

The complex head movements in Crane Feeding on pages 146–147 are led by the chin. The ren mai—the yin half of the microcosmic orbit (see pages 28–29)—terminates at the chin, while the du or yang meridian ends at the hard palate, or roof of the mouth. During Crane Feeding, focus your mind on the tongue, which links the two. Your head moves in a circle, with your chin leading. As you complete the circle you arch your head back,

tucking your chin in, and pull your chin and your head up. This brings Qi to the top of your head and down again to your chin. As you pull up, you bend your knees and lower your pelvis, giving your spine a good stretch. You circle your chin three times, sitting a little lower each time. Remember not to sink too far down as you make the first two circles. As you begin the third, you should be in a semisquatting position.

Minimal movements

You rise to a standing position during Craning the Neck on page 143. Your head leads, lifting first to the right, then to the left. The movement is effected by extending the muscles at the side of the neck in a movement so small it scarcely merits being called a stretch. It looks somewhat as if the side of the head were being lifted by a string attached to the temple. With each head movement you straighten your legs and lift your hips a little. As long as you do not lift too far each time, the sixth lift will bring you to a standing position.

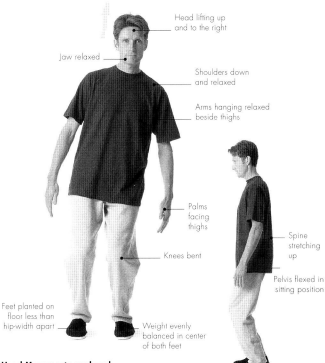

Head lifting up
and to the right

Jaw relaxed

Shoulders down
and relaxed

Arms hanging relaxed
beside thighs

Palms
facing
thighs

Knees bent

Feet planted on
floor less than
hip-width apart

Weight evenly
balanced in center
of both feet

Spine
stretching
up

Pelvis flexed in
sitting position

Head Movements analyzed

This illustration shows the positioning of all parts of the
body in the squatting position in which you finish Crane
Feeding on page 142. The arrow indicates the
direction you move your head in step 1 of Craning the
Neck, which follows it. Your head moves left and right
twice more, and with each movement left or right you
straighten your legs and lift your hips a little. By step 6,
you are standing upright.

Crane Feeding analyzed

Start the head movements in
Crane Feeding on page 142
by projecting your chin
forward, then push it down,
tuck it in, and pull it up to draw
a circle with your chin.

SECRETS OF QIGONG

145

HIP CIRCLES

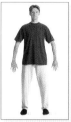

The last movements on pages 144–145 raise you from a semisquat to an upright stance. You stretch your arms up as if lifting energy you have gathered to your head, and tipping it into the third eye. Then the form continues its theme of stretching and moving the spine with an exercise that involves circling the pelvis and so rotating the lumbar spine. The massaging effects of these movements are followed by a self-massage to ease low back pain resulting from poor posture and lack of exercise.

Start position
Begin with your feet a little less than hip-width apart, knees and elbows slightly bent, hands by your sides, palms facing thighs.

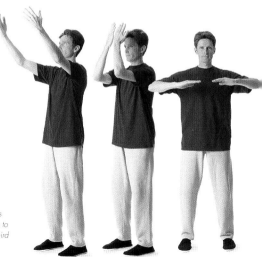

The Third Eye
Raise your hands to your brow, extending your arms and turning your palms up to repeat steps 1–3 of the Third Eye on pages 126–127.

Hip Circles

1 *Move your elbows and pull your hands out to the sides of your head, then lower your hands, palms turning down, to the lower dantian, and resume the start position. Then bending your elbows, draw your hands in until the outsides of your thumbs touch your hip bones.*

2 *Keeping your hands in contact with your body, roll them around your hips until the thumbs touch behind you and the fingers overlap. Press the backs of your hands against the small of your back.*

3 *Bending your knees a little, press the backs of your hands against your back, and rotate your hips clockwise three times, then change direction, circling them three times counterclockwise.*

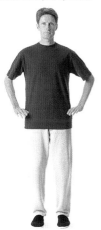

Finish and move on

Finish by moving your hands apart a little, while keeping them pressed against your lower back, and massaging your back by making three small circles with the backs of your hands rubbing against the base of your spine.

Self-Massage

Rotating your hips while pressing against the lower spine with the backs of your hands in hip circles on pages 146–147 massages the kidneys. The result is to increase the blood supply to them, speeding the elimination of waste products from the body, and increasing the circulation of blood and lymph to these organs. Hip rotations also feel good since they have a soothing effect on the major nerve center at the base of the spine.

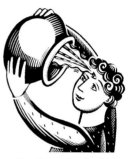

Nourishing the yin dang

As you begin the Third Eye on page 146, imagine yourself lifting a great cauldron of Qi up above your head and tipping it so that a stream of glowing energy pours from its lip into the third eye or yin dang energy center in your brow.

Easing low back pain

The beneficial effects of this exercise depend on smoothly flowing movements. At the beginning, the hands slide around the body from the front to the back without losing contact; and the hip rotations change seamlessly from clockwise to counterclockwise, and merge without a break into the circular movements of the massaging hands.

Poor posture puts a strain on the spine and neglecting to exercise weakens the muscles that hold it erect. The result is aching and often more acute pain in the lower part of the back. Massaging the back directly, using the simple self-massage technique illustrated opposite, relieves these aches and pains and stimulates the blood supply to the spine. An alternative way of massaging the small of the back is shown on page 213. Techniques such as do-in or brisk patting, shown on pages 204–205, and gentle stroking as on page 209, improve circulation to the spine.

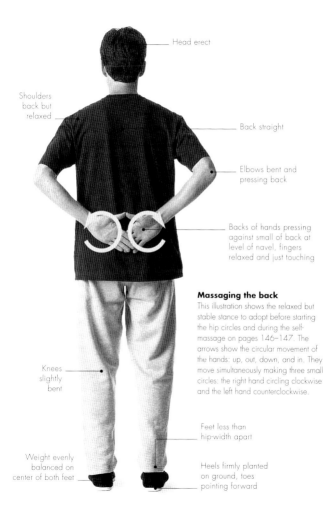

Head erect

Shoulders back but relaxed

Back straight

Elbows bent and pressing back

Backs of hands pressing against small of back at level of navel, fingers relaxed and just touching

Massaging the back

This illustration shows the relaxed but stable stance to adopt before starting the hip circles and during the self-massage on pages 146–147. The arrows show the circular movement of the hands: up, out, down, and in. They move simultaneously making three small circles: the right hand circling clockwise and the left hand counterclockwise.

Knees slightly bent

Feet less than hip-width apart

Weight evenly balanced on center of both feet

Heels firmly planted on ground, toes pointing forward

KNEE ROTATIONS

Two exercises for loosening the knees follow the hip circles on the preceding pages. Rotating the knees mobilizes the knees, which carry all the weight of the upper body. Constantly in use, commonly abused, yet rarely if ever exercised to maintain their strength and preserve their flexibility, the knee joints require surgery more often than any other joint in the body. Scissors, the second of the two exercises, flexes and extends the muscles of the thighs and hips, which turn the legs inward and outward.

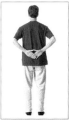

Start position
Begin with your feet a little less than hip-width apart, knees slightly bent, elbows bent, and the backs of your hands against the small of your back.

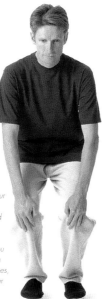

Knee Rotations
1 *Keeping your palms against your body, move your hands down behind you to your thighs, and then around to your knees, bending your legs and lowering your hips as you do so. Stop when you get close to a sitting position with your hands on your knees, and place the centers of your palms over your kneecaps.*

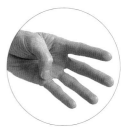

Contain your Qi
At the beginning of step 1, place the tip of each thumb on the pad beneath the fourth finger, and keep it there as you slide your hands from your lower back, down your buttocks and thighs, and around to your knees. Release your thumbs as you place your palms on your kneecaps.

2 Transfer your weight forward, lift your heels, and pivoting on the balls of your feet, move your knees clockwise in a large circle. Make the circle as large as you can, and follow it with two more rotations.

3 Keeping your palms on your knees, circle your knees three times counterclockwise, pivoting on the balls of your feet. Make the circles as large as you can.

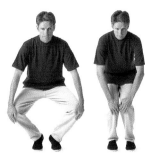

Scissors

With your knees still bent in the squatting position and your heels raised, open your knees wide and close them again three times in succession, keeping your palms on your kneecaps.

Exercising the Legs

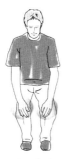

Warming the knees

Rub your hands together to generate Qi before beginning the knee rotations. Your thumb placed on the pad beneath your fourth finger contains warm Qi in your hand while you move it down to your knees. Feel it radiate from your hands into your knees when you place your palms on your kneecaps.

Knee Rotations and Scissors on page 150–151 are simple movements, but together they exercise the entire leg from the hip joint to the foot. Sitting without the support of a chair is one of the best ways of exercising muscles hidden deep in the pelvis which bend the hip joint. Scissors bends and stretches groups of small

muscles that move the thigh in toward the center of the body and away from it. Knee rotations stretch the muscles that bend and straighten the knees. Squatting and pivoting on the balls of the feet work the ankle joints and the muscles of the legs and feet.

Stimulating energy flow

Circling the knees not only loosens the knee joints but it also stimulates the flow of Qi around the body. Before beginning the knee circles you capture some of the energy you generated when circling your hips and massaging your back on pages 146–147, and carry it in the palms of your hands down to your knees.

To be effective, both exercises need to be carried out vigorously. Make the three knee circles as big as you can, and when opening and closing your legs in the scissors movement you need to move your knees wide apart. Rising onto the balls of your feet and lifting your heels help you make bigger circles and enable you to balance while moving your legs in and out.

Knee Rotations analyzed

Check the points detailed in this illustration to make sure you are properly balanced to circle your knees as shown on pages 150–151. The center of the circle you make with your knees needs to be over the balls of your feet, not over your heels, so check that your weight is forward. Tuck in your seat for better balance, stretch your spine up, and align your head with it.

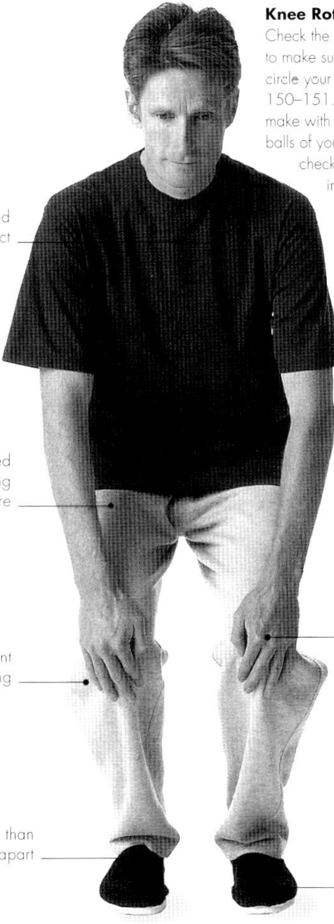

Trunk and head erect

Hips flexed into sitting posture

Knees bent and circling

Palms of hands placed on kneecaps

Feet less than hip-width apart

Balls of feet pivoting

SPINAL STRETCH

Part 3 ends with an upward stretch which exercises your legs, your back, and your neck. Follow with an upward stretch to bring invigorating Qi to the yin dang or third eye energy, then lower your hands in a gathering movement to finish.

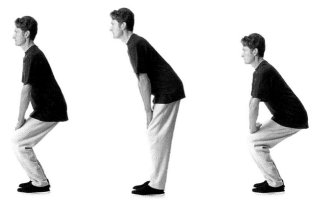

Spinal stretch

1 *You ended step 2 of Scissors on page 151 in a sitting position, balancing on the balls of your feet, hands on knees, palms over kneecaps. Now drop your heels to the ground, move your hands up onto your thighs, and turn them inward so your fingers rest on your inner thighs just above the knees.*

2 *Fix your gaze on a point at eye level, and keeping your hands on your thighs above your knees, move your weight to the balls of your feet, and straighten your legs. Relax your jaw and let your mouth open as your weight comes forward.*

3 *Bend your legs again—a little more than last time—and drop your hips fractionally closer to the floor. Keeping buttocks tucked in and head high, straighten your legs a third time.*

Repeat and finish

Repeat step 3 once, then bend your knees and lower your pelvis to a squatting position.

The Third Eye

Raising your hands from your thighs lift your arms, straightening your legs at the same time. As your hands reach your head, turn the palms toward you and repeat steps 1–3 of the Third Eye on pages 126–127.

Gathering In

1 At the end of the Third Eye, move your hands, palms turned to the ground, down the front of your body. As they reach the level of the dantian, bend your knees and drop your hips into a squatting position once again. At the same time, slice your hands sideways through the air in front, then down, turning the palms to face you, as if you were gauging the size of a huge ball of Qi.

2 Bringing your hands close into your body, bend your elbows and move your arms up as if lifting the ball of Qi to hold it against the lower dantian. Finish in the classic stance with your hands slightly cupped, palms turned up, opposite the lower dantian, feet parallel, and eyes directed ahead.

Finish

The spinal workout that began with Crane Feeding on page 142 ends here with a vigorous stretch that extends from the hamstrings at the backs of the thighs to the top of the spine. You squat as if into a chair, bending your legs and dropping your hips, put your hands on your lower thighs, and straighten your legs. This exercise opens the lower back and stretches legs and spine, emphasizing the link between upper and lower body.

Drawing to a close

From the squat you straighten your legs and your trunk and lift your arms to bring fresh Qi up to the head and tip it into the third eye or brow center. This is the third appearance of the Third Eye in Part 3 of the form, but each time it appears, it starts from a different point. Here, you lift your hands from the knees.

You complete each part of the form in the classic QiGong standing posture, focusing your mind quietly on the Qi you have gathered and are

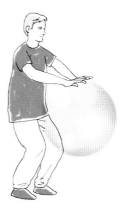

Gathering Qi

As you lower your hands in the final movement on page 155, imagine they encounter a huge ball of Qi and immediately gather it in to hold it against the dantian.

holding in your palms just opposite the lower dantian, which lies just below the navel. Each ending is slightly different, however, and here you circle your hands out in front of you to gather a huge ball of Qi and bring it in to hold it close to your body.

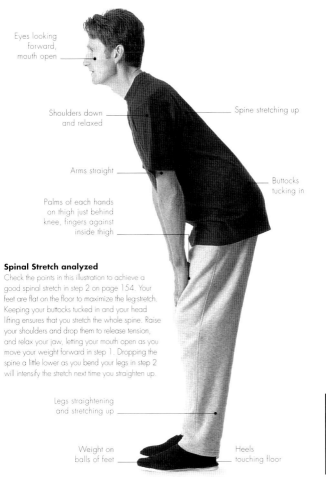

Eyes looking forward, mouth open

Shoulders down and relaxed

Spine stretching up

Arms straight

Buttocks tucking in

Palms of each hands on thigh just behind knee, fingers against inside thigh

Spinal Stretch analyzed

Check the points in this illustration to achieve a good spinal stretch in step 2 on page 154. Your feet are flat on the floor to maximize the leg-stretch. Keeping your buttocks tucked in and your head lifting ensures that you stretch the whole spine. Raise your shoulders and drop them to release tension, and relax your jaw, letting your mouth open as you move your weight forward in step 1. Dropping the spine a little lower as you bend your legs in step 2 will intensify the stretch next time you straighten up.

Legs straightening and stretching up

Weight on balls of feet

Heels touching floor

WHITE CRANE PART 4

A replenishing of Qi through the third eye makes an appropriate start to a succession of vigorous whole-body movements that leave you feeling energized. Bouncing the Qi on pages 162–171 is a complex sequence that may take time to learn but is great fun to practice. You bounce lightly on one leg while making wavelike motions with your arms and hands in time to your body's up-and-down movements, or flapping your arms like a bird taking off into the air. Toward the end, your fingers form the magic wand ready to direct energy strongly outward. And you finish by collecting new Qi and pouring it into the third eye, your palms making a triangle with your brow and actively pressing the Qi into the energy center in a spiraling movement. Part 4 demands all the timing and coordination of a dance to be effective. It stimulates all major body systems— the breathing, the circulation of blood and lymph, and the central nervous system—so it leaves you fully alert.

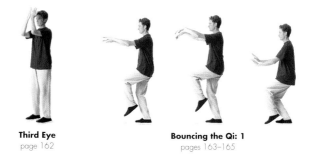

Third Eye
page 162

Bouncing the Qi: 1
pages 163–165

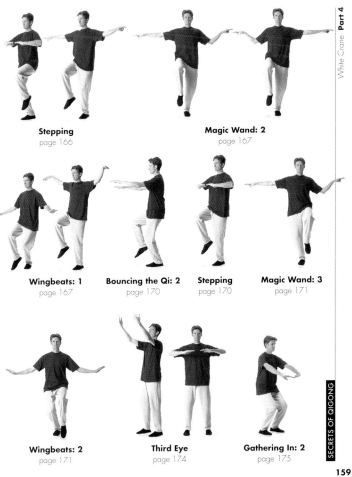

Stepping
page 166

Magic Wand: 2
page 167

Wingbeats: 1
page 167

Bouncing the Qi: 2
page 170

Stepping
page 170

Magic Wand: 3
page 171

Wingbeats: 2
page 171

Third Eye
page 174

Gathering In: 2
page 175

Internal Systems

Subtly but effectively you continue to work on the hips and legs through Part 4, but you focus so strongly on coordinating the rhythmic movements of your arms and body that you scarcely notice it. Bouncing the Qi exercises key muscles buried so deep in the abdomen you rarely are aware of them. Collectively called the iliopsoas, they bend and rotate the thigh, and one of their functions is to allow you to raise one leg off the floor. These are the muscles of balance, and when they are weak you are likely to wobble. Exercising them as you do in Bouncing the Qi strengthens them and improves your stability. Regular practice once you have progressed to the stage where you can perform the arm movements with your toes lifted high off the floor keeps the iliopsoas strong.

Balance is a major theme in Part 4; you balance every one-sided move by repeating it on the other. Having completed a set of movements while standing on the left leg, you step forward, transfer your weight to the right leg, and

The microcosmic orbit
By now you should be finding it easier to use the power of your mind to guide the circulation of Qi around the microcosmic orbit, shown here. Guide it for two or three circuits before moving on.

repeat the movements with the left leg lifted. This form strives to achieve an equilibrium between movements on the left and right, front and back, down and up, to balance the flows of energy into and out of your body. Pushing to the sky on one side attracts energy of a particular type into only one part of your body. Balancing that energy is an aspect of almost every movement in the form. The form also tries to maintain a balance between visualization to help achieve the movements, and losing yourself in dreaminess. This is achieved by keeping your eyes open as you practice, even while exercising your imagination, but keeping them in soft focus on the middle distance. That encourages the circulation of Qi. And at times an instruction to focus—on the palms of your hands in step 2 of Third Eye, for instance—exercises your vision and your alertness.

Laogong center

Standing meditation

Even when you know the form thoroughly you always pause for a minute at the beginning of each part to follow the pathway of the Qi around the body with your mind. By now you should be able to lead its branching across the shoulders and down the arms to the laogong center in the palms of the hands.

BOUNCING THE QI: 1

Part 4 of the form opens with a series of wavelike arm movements, but unlike Undulating Arms at the beginning of Part 1, these movements are more fluid. There is also more emphasis on balance, for you rest all your weight on one leg and use it as a flexible base on which to bounce rhythmically while moving your arms and hands up and down. Touching the floor with the toes of the opposite foot helps you keep your balance until you can bounce the Qi with one leg lifted into the air.

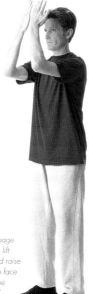

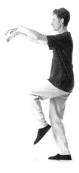

Achieving balance

Keep your left toes touching the floor for balance at first, then practice lifting them just clear of the floor as you straighten your right leg on the rebound in step 3. Eventually, you will be able to bounce with your foot lifted as high as 18 inches (45 centimeters) from the ground.

Third eye

From the standing posture on page 161, feet hip-width apart, you lift your hands from your sides and raise your arms, turning the palms to face up, and repeat steps 1–3 of the Third Eye on pages 126–127.

Bouncing the Qi: 1

1 Sweep both arms up in front of you to shoulder height, finishing with elbows straight and hands, palms down, stretching forward. As you do so, transfer all your weight to the right leg and foot, and bend your left knee, pointing the foot down toward the floor.

3 Now lift your shoulders, then your elbows, and let your wrists and hands sweep up to shoulder level. At the same time, straighten your right leg to raise your hips and lift your left toes clear of the floor.

2 Drop your shoulders, then your elbows, allowing your arms and wrists to sink down to the level of the dantian. As your arms move, bend your right knee a little to drop your hips closer to the floor.

Repeat and move on

Repeat steps 2 and 3 twice, so that your body bounces gently in time with the rhythmic, wavelike movements of your arms and hands. On the last upswing, straighten your arms and hands to return to step 1.

Balance and Movement

Bouncing the Qi energizes you, body and mind. It wakes you up because it activates your internal Qi, getting it moving and spreading it through your whole body. The arm movements are livelier and less subtle than those on pages 86–87. Rather than undulate, your arms make larger, looser movements, and bouncing on one leg makes your Qi move up and down, boosting its circulation. You need to drop your pelvis firmly to wake the Qi, rebounding lightly upward afterward.

Practicing regularly improves your balance. Positioning your weight correctly is the first essential. Beginners often start by moving some weight to the right foot, but that is not enough Imagine a heavy pillar descending from your head, through your right shoulder and your right hip, and down your right leg. You need to transfer all your weight from the left side of your body to the right so your center of gravity is in the middle of your right foot. This grounds you firmly, so that when you bend your left knee and point the foot, you need

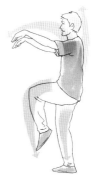

Waves of energy

Imagine waves of Qi washing through your body to awaken all your senses— their crests riding up your spine and into your head, along each arm to the fingers, and rolling down from the lower dantian to your feet and through them into the Earth.

make only small adjustments to balance yourself: stretch your spine and head up as if they were being lifted lightly from above, tuck your buttocks in, and fix your gaze on a point at eye level. Practicing strengthens the muscles of your hips, abdomen, and legs, which keep you upright and balanced.

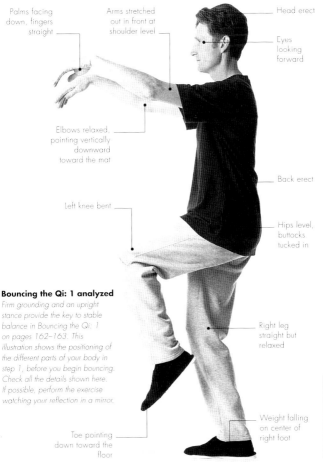

Palms facing down, fingers straight

Arms stretched out in front at shoulder level

Head erect

Eyes looking forward

Elbows relaxed, pointing vertically downward toward the mat

Back erect

Left knee bent

Hips level, buttocks tucked in

Bouncing the Qi: 1 analyzed

Firm grounding and an upright stance provide the key to stable balance in Bouncing the Qi: 1 on pages 162–163. This illustration shows the positioning of the different parts of your body in step 1, before you begin bouncing. Check all the details shown here. If possible, perform the exercise watching your reflection in a mirror.

Right leg straight but relaxed

Weight falling on center of right foot

Toe pointing down toward the floor

FLYING ENERGY

In Bouncing the Qi: 1 you bounced on the right leg, and now you move your weight to the left side of the body, and bend and straighten your left leg. As you change from your right leg to your left, you take a step, and that involves changing the orientation of your arms. First you make your hand into a magic wand and repeat the arm movements shown on pages 118–119, but with your arms stretched out to the sides. Then you make wavelike movements of your shoulders, arms, and hands, which imitate the flapping wings of a bird in flight.

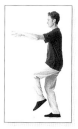

Start position
Stand on your right leg, left knee raised, arms swept up in front to shoulder height, palms facing down.

Stepping
1 *Bend your elbows to bring your arms to your chest, palms down, fingers straight, thumbs parallel to ribs, and step forward with your left foot, dropping the heel to the ground first.*

2 *Transfer all your weight to your left leg, and bend it slightly, dropping your pelvis toward the floor. Leading with the fourth finger of each hand, arc both arms out to the sides as in the breaststroke, keeping the palms of your hands facing down. Then lift your right knee and point the foot, touching the toes to the ground.*

Magic Wand: 2

1 As the stepping nears completion, bend your third and fourth fingers to your palms, and hold them with your thumbs to form the magic wand with your index and second fingers. Relaxing your left shoulder and dropping the elbow, pull your left hand down and in toward you.

2 In one flowing movement, straighten your left elbow to push your arm outward, while relaxing your right shoulder and elbow to pull your right hand toward you. Then straighten your right elbow to push the right hand out, while pulling your left hand in again.

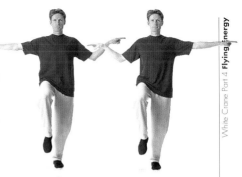

Repeat and move on

Keeping your elbows relaxed, your arms at shoulder height, and your fingers pointing out to the sides, repeat step 2 twice, making smooth, undulating movements with your arms, then release the magic wand, returning to your position at the end of Stepping.

2 Lift your shoulders and your elbows, letting your arms sweep up, followed by your hands. At the same time, straighten your left knee, raising your pelvis and lift your right toes clear of the floor.

Repeat and move on

Repeat steps 1 and 2 twice, beating your outstretched arms up and down like those of a bird in flight, your body bouncing gently in time with their rhythmic movements. After the last rebound, begin steadying your hands and arms ready to move on to Bouncing the Qi: 2 on page 170.

Wingbeats: 1

1 Drop your shoulders, then your elbows, letting your wrists and hands sweep down to the level of your dantian. As your arms move, bend your left knee to drop your hips and your right toes closer to the floor.

Improving Coordination

Coordination is especially important in Part 4 exercises, which involve moving arms and legs, hands and feet simultaneously and in different ways. It helps to imagine a connecting thread of Qi between parts of the body that are moving in tandem. For example, in step 1 of Bouncing the Qi: 1 on page 163, imagine a thread wound around your arms and tied to your left knee. As your arms sweep up to shoulder height, they pull the knee up. As you move into stage 2 of the exercise on page 166, your arms close in toward your chest as you step with your left foot, and they rest parallel with your collar bones as you lower your heel to the ground.

Rhythmic bouncing

Wingbeats: 2 on page 167 is a test of your coordination skills, since you bounce down and up on your left leg, while you raise and drop both arms. Concentrate on moving your shoulders and elbows, and your wrists and hands will follow, flapping like wings. It is

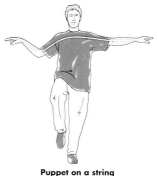

Puppet on a string
*The arms need perfect coordination:
as you pull one hand in toward you,
the other is pushing out.*

important to realize that although your bent right knee and the downward-pointing right foot lower and lift, you power their movements by bending and straightening your left leg, on which you stand. However, although you remain standing on your left leg all through Magic Wand: 2, you do not bend and straighten it in time to your arm movements. When you lift your right knee and foot at the start, they remain lifted through the exercise and on into Bouncing the Qi: 3 on page 170.

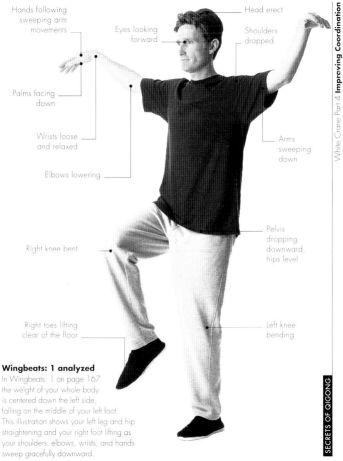

Hands following
sweeping arm
movements

Head erect

Eyes looking
forward

Shoulders
dropped

Palms facing
down

Arms
sweeping
down

Wrists loose
and relaxed

Elbows lowering

Pelvis
dropping
downward,
hips level

Right knee bent

Right toes lifting
clear of the floor

Left knee
bending

Wingbeats: 1 analyzed
In Wingbeats: 1 on page 167
the weight of your whole body
is centered down the left side,
falling on the middle of your left foot.
This illustration shows your left leg and hip
straightening and your right foot lifting as
your shoulders, elbows, wrists, and hands
sweep gracefully downward.

BOUNCING THE QI: 2

This begins with a second transfer of weight, from the left side to the right, and a step with your right foot. Stepping also involves changing the orientation of your arms from front to sides, from bouncing to flying energy, in which you imitate the beating wings of a bird in flight. You go on to repeat the movement sequence on pages 166–167, but standing on your right leg.

Start position
Stand on your left leg, right knee bent, arms out to the sides, palms facing down.

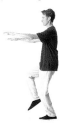

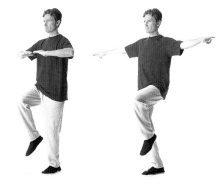

Bouncing the Qi: 2
Feel around an imaginary horizon with your fingers until both arms stretch out in front, palms facing down. Then, repeat the wavelike arm movements of steps 2 and 3 of Bouncing the Qi: 1 on page 163 three times, standing on your left leg. Finish on an upswing.

Stepping
1 Bend your elbows out to the sides, bringing your hands in to your chest, palms down, fingers straight, thumbs parallel to ribs. Then step forward with your right foot, dropping the heel to the ground first.

2 Transfer your weight to your right leg and bend the knee, dipping your pelvis toward the floor. Leading with the forefinger of each hand, arc both arms out to the sides, keeping your palms facing down. Then lift your left knee and point your foot, toes touching the ground.

Magic Wand: 3

As the stepping movement reaches completion, form the magic wand with your hands, relax your left shoulder, and pull your left hand in toward you. Then, repeat step 2 of Magic Wand: 2 on page 167 three times, keeping your right leg slightly bent and your left knee lifted, your left foot pointed and your toes touching the ground. Finally, release the magic wand and steady your arms.

Wingbeats: 2

With your arms still stretching out to the sides, lift your shoulders and elbows, bend your left knee to drop your hips, and repeat steps 1 and 2 of Wingbeats: 2 on page 167 three times. Your arms move rhythmically, imitating the flapping wings of a bird in flight, while your body bounces down and up in time with them.

Finish and move on

Finish Wingbeats: 2 on an upswing, then straighten your arms and steady your hands ready to move to the final movement sequences of Part 4 on page 174.

Smooth Transitions

In Bouncing the Qi on pages 162–171 each movement and each sequence must flow smoothly and merge seamlessly into the next. Once you have learned the sequence of actions your arms must make, you need to practice merging the movements of your arms, hands, hips, and legs, to make them flow gracefully. To achieve this, the shoulders must power them as shown in Magic Wand on pages 118–119. In Wingbeats on pages 167 and 171 your arms move more loosely and dynamically, but they must flow gracefully. To achieve this, lift or lower your shoulders first, then the elbows, but leave the wrists loose and relaxed enough to follow their own route, leading the hands. As you drop your shoulders and elbows, your arms sweep down, reaching the level of the dantian before the hands arrive there. As you raise your shoulders and elbows, your wrists sweep up, your hands following. Your arms have already started their next downward sweep before the hands reach shoulder level.

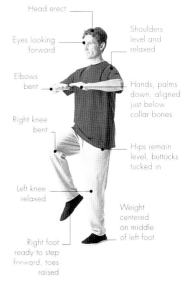

Head erect

Eyes looking forward

Shoulders level and relaxed

Elbows bent

Hands, palms down, aligned just below collar bones

Right knee bent

Hips remain level, buttocks tucked in

Left knee relaxed

Weight centered on middle of left foot

Right foot ready to step forward, toes raised

Stepping analyzed

The stepping movement on page 170 helps you make a smooth transition from balancing on the left leg to balancing on the right. As long as your weight is firmly grounded at the end of Bouncing the Qi 2, your hips level, and your right knee lightly lifted, you can step smoothly forward with your right foot and place your heel gently down on the ground.

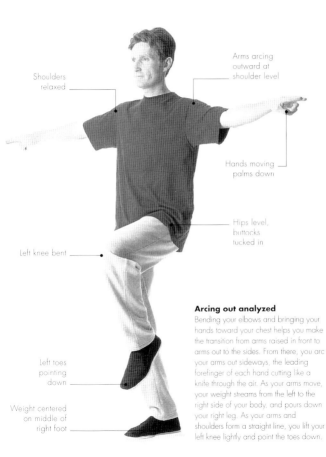

Shoulders relaxed

Arms arcing outward at shoulder level

Hands moving palms down

Hips level, buttocks tucked in

Left knee bent

Left toes pointing down

Weight centered on middle of right foot

Arcing out analyzed

Bending your elbows and bringing your hands toward your chest helps you make the transition from arms raised in front to arms out to the sides. From there, you arc your arms out sideways, the leading forefinger of each hand cutting like a knife through the air. As your arms move, your weight streams from the left to the right side of your body, and pours down your right leg. As your arms and shoulders form a straight line, you lift your left knee lightly and point the toes down.

FINISH

The dynamic bouncing and flying movements of Part 4 are completed here as you step down with your left leg and send your hands down in a wide arc to rest at your sides. From there your movements merge into an upward stretch to press replenishing Qi into the Third Eye center in your brow. End Part 4 with the same gathering movement that ended Part 3, and a meditative pause for a minute or more in a standing posture.

Start position
You finished Wingbeats: 2 standing on your right leg, your left knee lifted, and arms partly stretched out just below shoulder level.

Third Eye
1 *Arc your hands down toward your thighs, and at the same time, lower your left foot to the floor about hip-width from your right foot. Continue moving the hands down to the sides of your body.*

2 *Lift your hands in front of you, turning the palms up, and repeat step 1 of the Third Eye on page 127, imagining yourself pouring liquid Qi into the yin dang.*

3 *Bend your elbows, bringing your hands closer to your brow to press Qi into the third eye, then follow step 3 of the Third Eye sequence on page 127.*

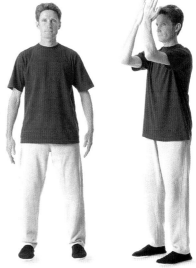

Gathering In: 2

1 As your hands reach the level of the dantian at the end of the Third Eye, repeat steps 1 and 2 of Gathering In on page 155, imitating the action of stooping to gather a huge ball of Qi and draw it toward you.

2 As your hands move up toward the lower dantian at the end of Gathering In, straighten your legs and lift your hips to finish in the classic stance with your hands slightly cupped, palms turned up opposite the lower dantian, feet parallel, and eyes directed ahead.

Energizing Exercise

The energetic sinking and raising of Qi while bouncing and flying through Part 4 activates its circulation so that you always feel energized at the end of the sequence. As you move rhythmically up and down on one leg, you enliven your Qi and wake your whole body up.

Role of breathing

Breathing plays a major part in this energizing process. Too great a focus on breathing can be distracting for a beginner, but at this stage in the form it can be helpful to become aware of the role it plays in making the movements develop. Breathing in before a vigorous movement has an inflating effect that helps it grow. Breathing out helps bring a movement to an end. Breathing out during exertion smooths the transition from one movement to another, emphasizing rhythm through the form and improving timing and coordination.

Dynamic movements use energy, so Part 4 of the form begins and ends by replenishing the body's internal store of

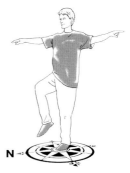

Footwork

Imagine yourself at the beginning of Part 4 standing at the center of a compass, facing north. Each time you step, first with your left foot, then with your right, you step further along the north-south meridian line.

energy through the yin dang. In its last movements you find a large ball of external Qi has arrived, and you gather it in to the lower dantian. Your motion is slowed by the natural rhythm of your breathing, and you rest, your upturned palms supporting the ball of Qi close to your lower dantian. Now you can enjoy a minute or more of stillness, contemplating the Qi you have garnered.

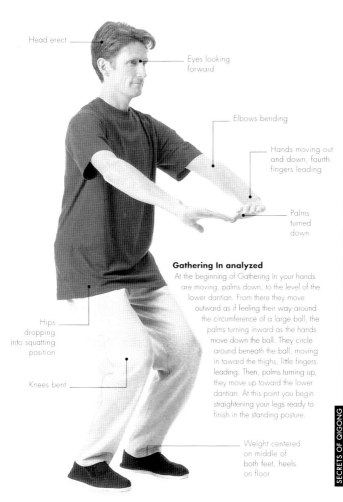

Head erect

Eyes looking
forward

Elbows bending

Hands moving out
and down, fourth
fingers leading

Palms
turned
down

Gathering In analyzed

At the beginning of Gathering In your hands
are moving, palms down, to the level of the
lower dantian. From there they move
outward as if feeling their way around
the circumference of a large ball, the
palms turning inward as the hands
move down the ball. They circle
around beneath the ball, moving
in toward the thighs, little fingers
leading. Then, palms turning up,
they move up toward the lower
dantian. At this point you begin
straightening your legs ready to
finish in the standing posture.

Hips
dropping
into squatting
position

Knees bent

Weight centered
on middle of
both feet, heels
on floor

WHITE CRANE PART 5

As you have progressed through the form you have performed many exercises that wash Qi down through the body from your shoulders and arms to your spine, hips, and legs, clearing spent energy and stale Qi, and relieving tension. Now it is time to work on the feet, and the central movements in Part 5 flex, stretch, and rotate each foot in turn. This final part of the form is a story of release, culminating with a kick with which you release physical tension and spent internal Qi. The kick is preceded by a turning movement, Looking Behind, which rotates the body from the hips. It also brings each hand in turn to point over the shoulder, palm facing up toward the ears, activating these organs' numerous meridians and energy points. And the foot rotations are followed by the exuberant Rainbow Circle, which rotates the whole body in a half circle, stretching the arms out to the sides, up to the sky, and down to the Earth, exercising the spine in four of its five directions of movement.

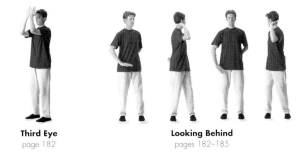

Third Eye
page 182

Looking Behind
pages 182–185

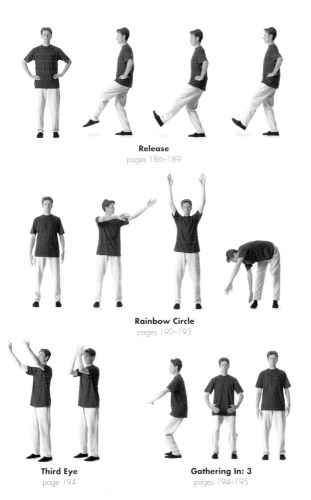

Release
pages 186–189

Rainbow Circle
pages 190–193

Third Eye
page 194

Gathering In: 3
pages 194–195

The Cosmic Link

Imagine your eyes sweeping through 180° to the left and then to the right in Looking Behind on pages 182–185, following the horizon out to the side and around behind you, sending your awareness outward, so you seem to step beyond yourself. The theme continues as you release stale Qi outward in the next exercise on pages 186–187, in a vigorous kick.

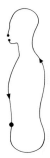

The web of life

Part 5 awakens your inner self to its link with the natural world beyond, to which it belongs. As you progress through each movement, think of yourself not as a separate entity divorced from nature but as an integral part of life. Love of nature was an ideal of the ancient Daoists, who saw it as the source of human happiness. The height of spirituality is, they believed, to achieve identification with nature in its entirety, in other words, with the universe.

Visualization exercises your mind, freeing it to travel beyond its present limits. Use the opportunity in the

The Microcosmic Orbit
As with the other four parts of the White Crane sequence, begin by visualizing the pathway of Qi around the microcosmic orbit. By this stage of the White Crane sequence you should be mentally atuned to thinking through three or four circuits to ensure you gain the most benefit from the exercises.

Rainbow Circle on pages 190–193 to send your consciousness out into the space beyond your hands, through the Earth's orbit and into the solar system. You stretch up past the stars out into deep space, and bend forward to reach into the cosmos, so that your moving hands encircle the universe, the source of all Qi. From this connection with the greater Qi, the Third Eye on page 194 reestablishes the connection with your personal Qi and the dantian, and the standing meditation that completes the form is an opportunity to calm your spirit and return to the reality of your personal existence.

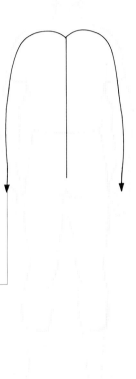

Laogong center

Standing meditation

Before you begin the movements of the final part of the form, stand for a minute or more generating a sense of the microcosmic orbit revolving like the wheel of life within your body, leading the Qi up the spine to branch across your shoulders and along your arms to your palms, ready to replenish the upper dantian energy center.

LOOKING BEHIND

Part 5 of the form begins with a replenishment of internal energy through the Third Eye and a series of three turns left and right. These turns rotate the whole body from the ankles to the head, exercising the hips and the waist. And as you turn your head, you look back out of the corner of your eyes, exercising and strengthening your peripheral vision—your ability to see out of the corners of your eyes—as well as affirming awareness of all that lies behind you.

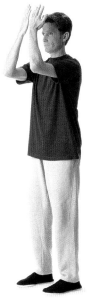

Third eye

From the standing posture on page 181, lift your hands from your sides, turning the palms to face up and repeat steps 1–3 of the Third Eye on pages 126–127.

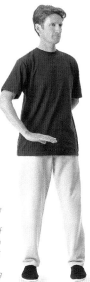

Looking behind

1 *As your left hand, palm turned down, reaches your waist in the last movement of the Third Eye, circle it round your hip, keeping the back of the hand and fingers in contact with your body, and rest it on your lower back at the level of the navel. Then follow with your upper body, turning to the left.*

2 As your hips, shoulders, neck, and head turn to the left, swivel your gaze leftward to look behind you out of the corners of your eyes. Meanwhile, lift your right hand, turn the palm to face up, and point the fingers back over your right shoulder.

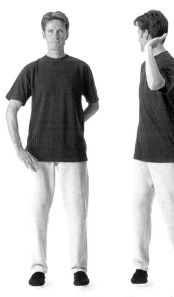

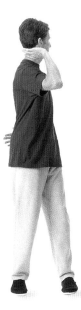

3 Release your right hand and move it down to your right hip. Follow the movement by turning your eyes, head, and upper body to face forward, while circling your right hand around your hip and behind you, keeping the back of the hand and the fingers in contact with your body.

4 Rest your right hand on top of your left and turn from the hips to the right, following with your eyes. As you turn, release your left hand and circle it around your left hip and up your chest to point over your left shoulder.

Repeat and finish

Turn to face forward while moving your left hand down from your shoulder to circle your left hip and rest it on your right hand. Then turn to the left while releasing your right hand, circling it around your hip, and raising it to point over your right shoulder. Repeat from step 3 twice, finishing on a right turn.

Turning

You begin Part 5 by looking back, turning to glimpse the part of the world, normally unseen, that lies behind you. These movements have layers of meaning, so that if you focus your awareness on the idea of looking back, you may find a new one each time you practice this exercise. Direct your mind back in time, perhaps to fathom the reasons for the origin and evolution of these movements. You might send it back into your personal time to contemplate the thoughts and actions that led you to these movements. Alternatively, think of the impact turning may have on the back of your body.

Rotating the spine

Your legs need to be straight, your buttocks tucked in, and your spine needs to be erect, stretching up from the sacrum at its base to your head, as you turn left and right. This enables you to rotate a little further, stretching your legs and hips and improving the flexibility of the muscles that control the rotation of the spine.

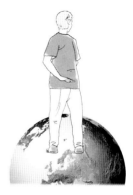

Beyond the horizon

When you turn to look over your left and right shoulders, imagine your eyes sweeping along the line of the horizon. As they move further around, you become aware of more and more of the world gradually emerging into your field of vision, until eventually you see beyond the horizon, out into the cosmos.

This exercise sharpens the peripheral vision and extends your visual range to almost 360°. Looking behind invites you to extend your awareness further, beyond your everyday horizons to see the whole world, and beyond that into the unknown forces of the universe.

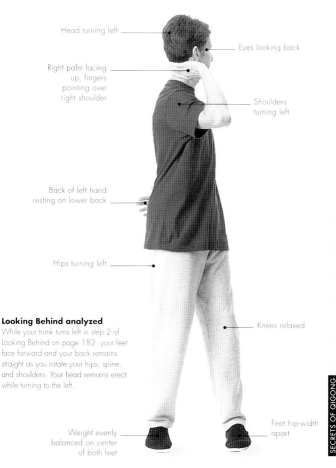

Head turning left

Eyes looking back

Right palm facing up, fingers pointing over right shoulder

Shoulders turning left

Back of left hand resting on lower back

Hips turning left

Knees relaxed

Looking Behind analyzed

While your trunk turns left in step 2 of Looking Behind on page 182, your feet face forward and your back remains straight as you rotate your hips, spine, and shoulders. Your head remains erect while turning to the left.

Weight evenly balanced on center of both feet

Feet hip-width apart

RELEASE

Having started by exercising the arms and hands, the form concludes its journey from head to toe through the body with vigorous kicks and foot rotations to exercise the joints, tendons, and muscles of the ankles and feet. Although they are in constant use, the feet are rarely exercised and these stretches and rotations help maintain the strength and elasticity of the joints, tendons, and muscles that control the movements of the feet. The kicks give a satisfying release of energy at the end of the form.

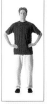

Start position
You finished Looking Behind on page 183 turning forward and bringing your hands to your hips, standing to begin Release with your feet hip-width apart.

1 *Transfer all your weight to the right side of the body and bend your left leg, lifting your foot clear of the floor. Centering your weight firmly on the middle of your right foot, pull your left foot back a little, point the toe, and kick, extending the leg and foot out in front.*

2 *Bend your left knee to withdraw your foot, turn the toes up and kick your left leg energetically forward and up, leading with the heel. Leave your lower leg comfortably extended after the kick.*

3 Now rotate your foot three times clockwise and three times counterclockwise. When you have completed the third rotation, leave your leg comfortably extended.

Repeat and finish
Repeat steps 1–3 twice more, then place your left leg on the floor. Then transfer your weight to the left side of your body, lift your right leg, and repeat steps 1–3 three times. Finish by placing your right leg on the floor and your hands by your sides.

Using the Feet

Internal Qi has worked its way down the body and built up in the feet, traditionally the site from which stale Qi leaves the body. Imagine yourself expelling bad Qi with a vigorous kick, first from your toes, then from your heels. It is important not to hold tension in your body, so kick fast and hard and feel the release after the split second of impact, but make the movement rhythmic and powerful, not jerky or aggressive. The foot rotations that follow the kicks massage your feet, relaxing the muscles and tendons.

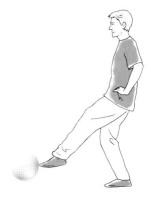

Releasing energy

As you lower your foot ready to kick, imagine accumulating excess internal energy in your foot and releasing it through the toes or the heel with a hard kick.

Maintaining balance

By now you should be able to lift your foot clear of the floor without supporting yourself. If you still wobble, check that all your weight is directed down the side of your body on which you stand, then tuck your buttocks in, stretch up, and gaze at some point straight ahead. Balance also guides the progress of the exercise, for you kick with your toe, then your heel, on the left side, then the right, and you circle your foot clockwise, then counterclockwise. And you try to achieve a balance between yang and yin after each kick, for although your hip and thigh muscles keep your knee lifted, you do not draw the foot back after the second kick with the heel. Instead, relax your knee and calf, letting leg and foot hang, still extended, from the raised knee.

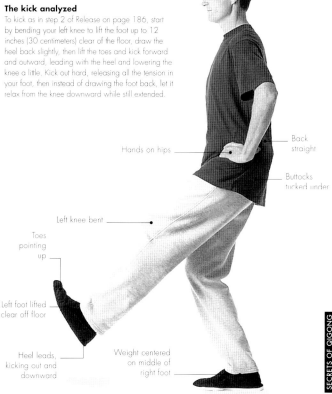

The kick analyzed

To kick as in step 2 of Release on page 186, start by bending your left knee to lift the foot up to 12 inches (30 centimeters) clear of the floor, draw the heel back slightly, then lift the toes and kick forward and outward, leading with the heel and lowering the knee a little. Kick out hard, releasing all the tension in your foot, then instead of drawing the foot back, let it relax from the knee downward while still extended.

Head erect

Hands on hips

Back straight

Buttocks tucked under

Left knee bent

Toes pointing up

Left foot lifted clear off floor

Heel leads, kicking out and downward

Weight centered on middle of right foot

RAINBOW CIRCLE

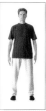

Imagine you are painting a huge rainbow that stretches across the sky and down under the Earth. This last dynamic exercise of the form involves the whole body as you stretch upward, swing out to the sides, and bend forward and down, painting the biggest rainbow you can imagine. It extends the spine in four directions, stretching and separating the vertebrae. It boosts the circulation of the blood, warming you up if you are cold. And it massages the internal organs, benefiting the liver especially.

Start position
Begin Rainbow Circle in the classic standing posture, your hands by your sides.

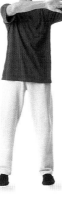

1 *Lift both hands from your hips and stretch them out to the left, turning the palms to face outward, so your right fingertips are close to the inside of your left elbow. Keep your hips and your head facing forward.*

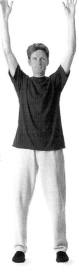

2 *Swing both arms up in an arc above your head, then around to the right, mirroring their position in step 1, and on downward.*

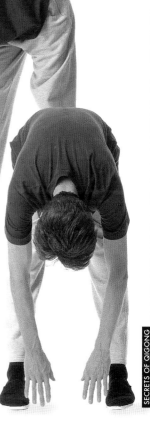

3 As your hands move down toward your right hip, drop your trunk forward, bending from the hips, keeping your legs straight but your knees relaxed, then sweep your arms up to the left again, inclining your body to the left as you rise.

Repeat and finish

Repeat steps 2 and 3 twice, then as you start the fourth upswing to the left, slow down, come to a stop, and reverse direction, swinging your arms back down, then around to the right. Make three full circles to the right, finishing on a downswing, bending forward with your fingers pointing toward your toes.

Whole Body Movement

The Rainbow Circle on pages 190–191 is a movement that leads Part 5 and the form toward its final conclusion. It completes the head-to-toe, inside-to-out stretching and exercising of the body by integrating the whole body in one dynamic movement. It completes the spreading of the Qi to all parts of the body, from your fingertips to your feet. It links your personal Qi to the greater Qi that unifies the cosmos.

The rainbow circle has the potential to extend you, physically and mentally, to link you with the cosmos. Draw the biggest circle you can and you grow taller as you extend your whole body upward. Imagine yourself reaching down into the Earth and you increase your spine's mobility as you bend to the left, forward, and to the right. Use this exercise to let your mind roam. Imagine your arms reaching up into the cosmos to the edges of the universe, your hands tracing the route of the Milky Way star pathway, and your fingers digging deep into the center of the Earth. Your hands move like the hands of a clock, through time, then backward, undoing time and setting it in reverse.

Circle into the cosmos
Imagine your hands reaching out beyond the edges of the Earth to touch a rainbow that extends out to the stars.

Rainbow Circle analyzed

As you reach into the Earth in step 3 of Rainbow Circle on page 191, bend forward from the hips (not from the waist) so your back is naturally straight as it hangs down. Remain relaxed—do not try to bend further than you comfortably can, just as far as you can go, reaching down with your arms and hands. Let your head hang. Your legs need to be straight, but keep your knees relaxed.

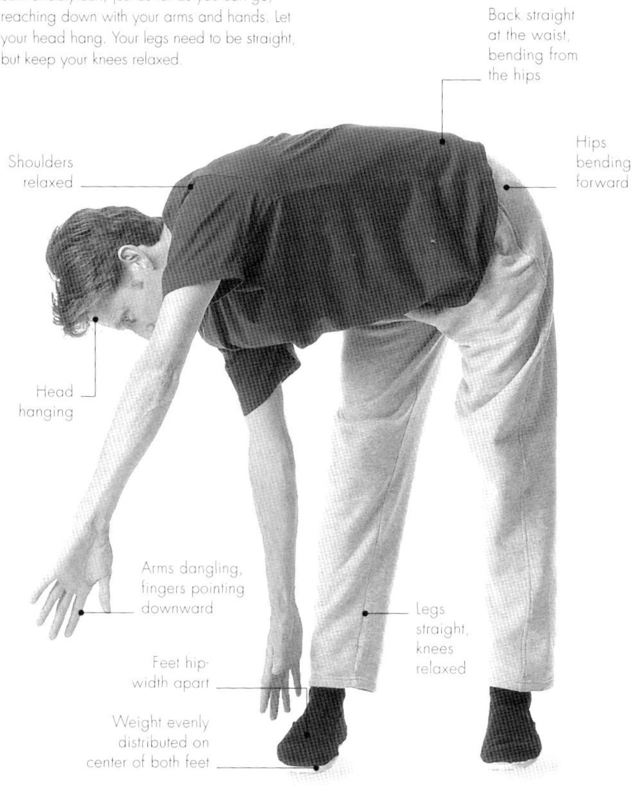

Back straight at the waist, bending from the hips

Hips bending forward

Shoulders relaxed

Head hanging

Arms dangling, fingers pointing downward

Legs straight, knees relaxed

Feet hip-width apart

Weight evenly distributed on center of both feet

FINISH

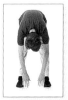

From the Rainbow Circle on pages 192–193, you squat down prior to lifting up and standing erect to empty the Qi you generated in the last exercise into the lower dantian. Then you repeat the standing meditation for the last time in the form, keeping your awareness clearly focused on the last movements and on the final gathering of the Qi. End the form on a note of peaceful contemplation so that you can carry a spirit of calm forward into your everyday life.

Start position
You finished the Rainbow Circle 2 on page 194 bending forward from the hips, arms and head hanging down toward your feet, knees relaxed.

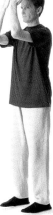

Third Eye
1 *Bending your knees, squat down a little before lifting from the hips. As you straighten your legs to stand upright, turn your hands palms up.*

2 *Keeping the palms facing up, raise your arms in front of you, lifting your hands to your head, and repeat steps 1–3 of the Third Eye on pages 126–127.*

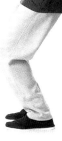

Gathering In: 3
1 *As your hands reach the level of the dantian at the end of the Third Eye, repeat steps 1 and 2 of Gathering In on page 155, imitating the action of stooping to gather a huge bull of Qi and draw it toward you.*

2 As your hands move up toward the lower dantian at the end of Gathering In: 3, straighten your legs and lift your hips to assume the classic stance with your hands slightly cupped, palms turned up opposite the lower dantian, feet parallel, and eyes directed ahead. Stand for a minute or more, consolidating the gathering of Qi into the dantian.

3 Drop your hands to your sides, palms facing your thighs. Experience a moment of stillness as you finish the last movement.

Final Moments

After connecting with external Qi, finish the form by reconnecting with your internal Qi through the lower dantian by performing the Third Eye for the last time. But as you lift your hands to this all-important energy center in your brow, you must rise from the final forward bend of the Rainbow Circle. To do this without straining your back, keep your legs well bent and your hips in a squatting position as you uncurl your spine and lift your shoulders, then raise your head, straightening your legs only when your hands reach shoulder height.

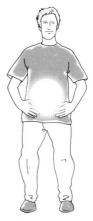

Treasure store
The movements of the form have accumulated a rich store of treasured energy for body and mind. Use the last moments of Part 5 to gather this treasure into the lower dantian so that as you leave, you know that it is safely stored there.

Completing the form

As you finish the Third Eye, approach the form's final moment with respect. Never drop your hands and dash off to begin something else. The movements that end each part of the form provide an opportunity to conserve energy, and so much Qi is held in the final moment that if you rush, you let it drain away. The effect is to weaken and tire you. Instead, stand for at least a minute with your hands palms turned partly up at the level of the dantian, and center yourself, quieting your spirit and gathering Qi into the dantian. Then, as you drop your hands, you can leave the Qi at the starting point of its route around the body, a store of energy to draw on.

Straightening up into Third Eye

Before raising your hands for the Third Eye, you squat and lift forward from the Rainbow Circle, straightening your legs as you rise. Keeping your feet firmly planted on the ground, raise your arms and your trunk as your legs straighten. Finish by lifting the crown of your head toward the sky and bringing your hands to chest level, turning the palms up.

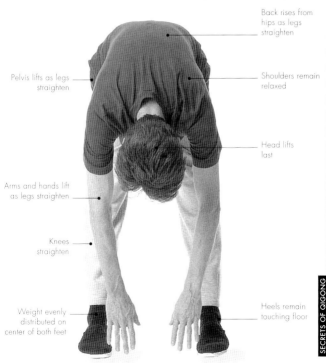

Back rises from hips as legs straighten

Shoulders remain relaxed

Pelvis lifts as legs straighten

Head lifts last

Arms and hands lift as legs straighten

Knees straighten

Weight evenly distributed on center of both feet

Heels remain touching floor

ENERGY
MANAGEMENT

QiGong is the art of managing Qi as a resource, so you always have enough for your daily needs. ～ This chapter looks at lifestyle and its effects on energy, and it explores ways of maximizing internal energy by extending QiGong beyond practice sessions into your daily life. ～ Allow QiGong to become your way of life and it can lift you physically and mentally, helping you handle problems you face in your work, in dealing with other people, and in coping with stress and aggression.

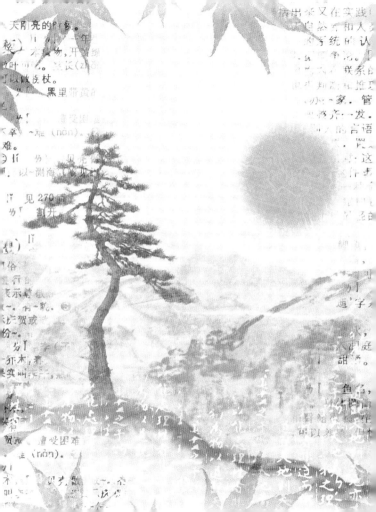

The QiGong Perspective

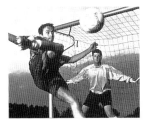

Sports training

QiGong makes you lighter and speedier, yet more powerful and more effective. You can relax under attack, or you can give a hefty tackle—and somehow, you are less likely to be injured.

Leave for work on Monday morning and for the first half of the day your mind feels as if it is stuck halfway through Sunday. You are uncoordinated and you forget things, and small issues can develop into problems. Practice the form for half an hour before setting off for work, and you will feel grounded and focused. You leave home feeling relaxed and mentally ready for anything. Physically, you feel good because you have exercised, so you are alert, alive, and altogether happier.

Training for life

Practicing QiGong regularly replenishes your treasured store of Qi, ensuring that it is not drained away by the energy demands of daily living, by eating too many meals made from preserved and processed food whose Qi content is low, and through skimping on sleep, which is important in replenishing Qi.

Regular QiGong practice benefits you mentally, making you feel more relaxed and self-confident. This helps you keep a balanced perspective on life so you are better able to deal with the daily challenges that cause negative stress. It quickly teaches you to apply QiGong in situations that cause a stress response. You become more aware of your body and learn to identify the tension rising in your shoulders, tightening your chest or stomach, or locking your jaw. You notice as your breathing rate quickens.

All QiGong movements may be practiced at any time in any situation, so you can use techniques such as deep breathing to counter tension. And you soon learn to employ the principles of QiGong to replace feelings of annoyance, disappointment, and anger with serenity. QiGong helps you clear your mind, be fully conscious of your feelings, and create a neutral space in which to handle them with awareness. It grounds and centers you, enabling you to think clearly.

The following pages show how QiGong techniques—breathing, movement, stretching, massage—may be applied to relieve difficult situations. All the techniques are widely applicable in any aspect of your life, to sports and hobbies, as well as work and home life. With time you can work out how to apply them to improve the quality of your life and to make yourself happier.

Overcoming stage fright

Stage fright is rising energy coming to a head as stress. QiGong can help you deal with it by teaching you to refocus—on abdominal breathing, for instance, or on the repetitive, rhythmic motions of Earth Wash (pages 70–71), or on active leg-swings (page 62). QiGong creates a place for the energy to go, enabling you to regain control.

DESKWORK

Breathing, stretching, and self-massage make a perfect antidote to the ill-effects of sitting at a desk for most of the working day. Prolonged sitting leads to physical and mental stagnation. The short program of QiGong techniques shown on these four pages wakes you up physically by working the muscles, getting oxygen into the blood, and speeding the circulation. Take five or ten minutes out of your working day and you will return to your desk more focused and alert, able to think faster and perform better.

Breathing

If you can, stand up to do this exercise, but if that is not possible remain seated at your desk and breathe in and out while lifting and lowering your arms.

Stand with your feet hip-width apart and your hands by your sides. Take a slow, deep breath and lift your arms out to the sides, turning the palms down, then stretch them up above your head. As your arms rise, bend your knees and squat down, feeling yourself lifted from the top of your head. Then lower your hands to your sides while straightening your legs. Repeat 3–5 times.

Massage your feet and exercise your ankles sitting at your desk. Do the exercise two or three times a day.

Take off your shoes and press the soles and heels of both feet into the floor, then release. Follow by lifting both heels and lowering them, then lift both forefeet and lower them. Repeat these movements nine times.

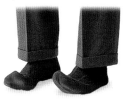

Moving

You can do a forward bend to stretch your spine while sitting at your desk—make a point of bending forward to pick things up from the floor. For the arm swings and shaking limbs you must be standing up. Perhaps you can find a quiet place during a break.

Forward bend

Stand erect with your feet hip-width apart, arms by your sides. Drop your head to your chest and slowly curl your spine forward, one vertebra at a time, into a forward bend. Drop as far as you comfortably can, then bend your knees, uncurl your spine, lift your head, and stand up.

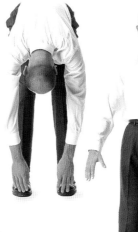

Arm swings

Stand with your feet hip-width apart, toes and heels on the floor, your arms hanging by your sides. Turning from the hips, rotate your spine to the right and back to the front, to the left and back to the front, swinging your arms loosely. Repeat for about 30 seconds.

Shaking limbs

Stand with your feet hip-width apart. Hold both arms a few inches from your body and shake your arms and your hands as if you were shaking off drops of water. Lift your right foot and shake that in the same way, then your left foot. Shake for 30 seconds, then rest.

Moving and Shaking

Energetic stretching, swinging, and shaking the limbs are the answer to the fatigue and sluggishness that will always set in if you work your mind for long periods without moving your body. They stimulate the circulation of blood, which brings oxygen to the brain and lymph, and clears wastes from the tissues, and they dispel tension.

Do-in, best described as a brisk patting, and anmogong, or self-massage, are techniques traditionally used to treat pain and illnesses. A technique for massaging the lower back, often a weak area in people who do sedentary work, is shown on page 149, and pinching the rims of the ears (see page 212) counters lethargy. Self-massage is effective in dispelling fatigue because stimulating certain acupressure points raises levels of mental alertness.

Even if you cannot leave your desk and take a break, you can still stretch, breathe deeply, and rub your head, neck, shoulders, back, and arms now and again while at your work station. Your work will certainly benefit.

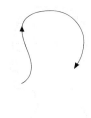

Head massage
Place the fingertips on the cheeks close to the jawline, close the eyes, and massage up to the forehead and back, across the scalp as if combing the hair with the fingers, and down to the back of the neck. Repeat about 3 times.

Program

This eight-minute program will restore your mental equilibrium and physical sense of well-being in the middle of the day or at the end, as you finish work.

1 Breathing (see page 202)   2 minutes
2 Arm swings (see page 203)   30 seconds
3 Forward bend (see page 203)   1 minute
4 Shaking limbs (see page 203) 30 seconds
5 Do-in (see page 205)   1 minute
6 Anmogong (see page 208)   1 minute
  – eye massage
  – head massage
7 Earth wash (see pages 70–71) 2 minutes

Do-in

Using the palms of first the right hand, then the left, briskly pat the whole arm from the shoulder down to the wrists, then the legs, the chest, and the middle to lower back, making firm slapping movements. The patting stimulates the acupressure points shown in the illustration on the right.

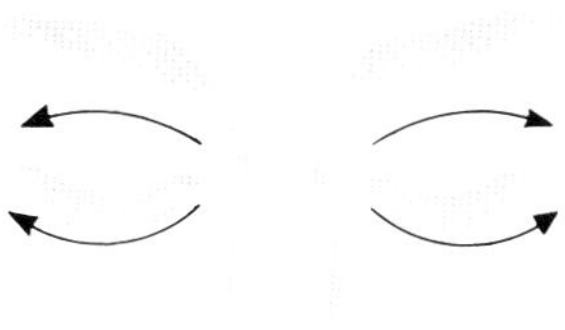

Eye massage

Place the tips of the middle fingers in the inner corner of each eye and lightly brush across the upper eyelids to the outer corners. Return to the inner corners and repeat, brushing across the lower eyelids. Repeat both movements about 20 times.

PARENTING AND CARING

If your work involves taking care of others, you need to find time each day for ten minutes' active relaxation, taking time to focus inward, on yourself and your own concerns and needs. Caretakers often spend time on their feet and their work may involve lifting and carrying, with consequent strain on the spine. This short exercise program involves calming breathing, total relaxation, and movements to mobilize the hip joints and stretch the legs, knees, ankles, and feet. In time this routine will increase your stamina.

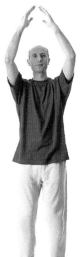

Breathing: 1

1 *Lie on the floor with your head and your spine in line, your knees on a cushion, and, if possible, your feet 6–12 inches (15–30 centimeters) higher than your hips.*

2 *Close your eyes, let your feet fall to either side, and place your hands, one on top of the other, on the lower dantian. Breathe rhythmically through the nose. As you breathe in, imagine your body filling with warm golden light; and as you breathe out, visualize all the tensions and annoyances of the day rushing out of your body. Lie, breathing gently, for about two minutes.*

Breathing: 2

1 *Stand with your feet hip-width apart, your hands by your sides. On a long slow in-breath, raise your arms out to the sides, turning your palms up until they touch above your head.*

2 *On a long, slow out-breath, and keeping your palms together, bend your elbows and lower your hands in front of your face and your trunk, separating them as they descend to the lower dantian. Lower them to your sides. Repeat three times.*

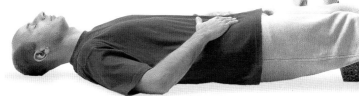

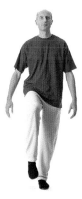

Moving

Looking after other people involves spending a lot of time on your feet, often standing still or walking short distances frequently. These exercises mobilize the hips, legs, and feet, stretching and bending them, moving the muscles, and getting the circulation going.

Foot circles

Repeat the foot rotations in Release on page 187, circling each foot three times clockwise and three times counterclockwise, first with your right leg, then with your left.

Wild Horse

Stand on your left leg, bend your right knee, lifting the foot clear off the ground, and circle the leg forward, down, back, and up like the pawing movement a horse makes, but without touching the ground. Repeat, circling the leg back, down, forward, and up. Now stand on your right leg, lift the left foot, and repeat the whole exercise circling the left leg.

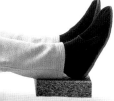

Kicks

Repeat the kicks in Release on pages 186–187, first with the toes pointed, then with the toes pointing up and leading with the heels. Kick first with the right leg, then with the left. Before you kick be sure of your balance, and kick vigorously but smoothly. As you kick, enjoy releasing any anger or pent-up aggression you may have built up as throughout the day.

Focus on Yourself

Caring for others, as a parent, a salesperson, a teacher, or a nurse can drain you. A ten-minute break is essential for you to recharge. You need time alone to banish negative energy and fatigue and to nurture yourself.

Spend the first two or more minutes in total relaxation. Lie on the floor, relax physically, and direct your mind to your breathing. Deepen each breath and follow its rhythm. Then concentrate on releasing doubts, frustrations, irritations, and other negative feelings with each exhalation filling your body with warm Qi on each inhalation. The Qi is golden, a protective color. It protects your inner self from the demands of others. Keeping that sense of inner self, think next about your outer self. Focus on the Qi flowing along your meridians as you exercise your hips, legs, and feet, stimulating blood and lymph to circulate, carrying nourishment to all your tissues.

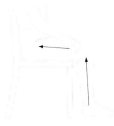

Anmogong

To stimulate the circulation of blood and lymph up the legs, against the force of gravity, massage upward, from ankle to knee, and from knee to hip. Make long, strong strokes with the palms and fingers, starting at the back of the legs and working around the sides to the front, for about two minutes.

To ease stiff knees, sit cross-legged on a chair, or on the floor, place your palms on your knees, and move them clockwise around the knee, opening and closing your hands to pinch and squeeze as you go, for about 30 seconds.

Finish by standing, palms facing down, feeling centerd and relaxed, and look around you. Take three deep breaths, stretching up and out on each inhalation. Your exhalations link you with the surrounding space, drawing you out and returning you to the world of others.

Clearing

Stroke your body from top to toe to clear stale Qi. Place both hands palms down on your head and stroke down your face and head to your chin and neck, down your torso from neck to hips, armpits to thighs, shoulder blades to buttocks. Then stroke down your legs from your thighs to your toes.

Program

After 10–12 minutes, this program of exercises from pages 206–209 will relax, then reinvigorate you.

1 Breathing: 1   2–4 minutes
2 Wild horse (see page 206)   30 seconds
3 Hip rotator (see page 207)   30 seconds
4 Kicks (see page 207)   30 seconds
5 Foot circles (see page 207)   30 seconds
6 Earth wash (see page 70–71) 1 minute
7 Anmogong (see page 208)
   – legs and feet massage   30 seconds
   – knee massage   30 seconds
   – clearing   1 minute
8 Breathing: 2 (see page 206) 30 seconds

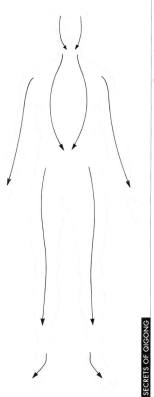

ON THE ROAD

Restricted movement usually limits the possibilities of exercise for drivers and also for their passengers in cars and on most other forms of transportation. Yet it also makes exercise a pressing need, for being confined in a small space adds to the tensions of any journey. QiGong offers a range of techniques to reduce stress for drivers and prevent it from rebuilding, to minimize the physical discomforts of sitting for long periods in cramped conditions, and to recover from its effect on mind and body.

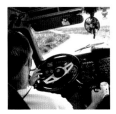

Breathing

Close your mouth, place the tip of your tongue against your upper teeth, and breathe in slowly. Hold the breath briefly, then open your lips slightly, let your tongue drop to the floor of your mouth, and take a long, slow exhalation. Repeat twice more, lengthening the out-breath each time. Repeat the three breathing cycles at regular intervals throughout the journey.

Sitting

The seats in many vehicles are poorly designed and induce sluggishness, especially on long journeys, which is dangerous for drivers. Adjusting your posture regularly while driving on highways, or during brief stops at traffic lights, keeps you alert.

1 *Place both feet flat on the floor if you can, place your hands on your knees or evenly on the steering wheel, relax your shoulders, look into the middle distance, and let all your body weight fall into the seat. Let the back of the seat support your spine.*

2 *Lift your head up, breathe deeply and rhythmically for about 30 seconds, and imagine the stresses of driving and traveling melting and pouring down through the seat and out onto the road.*

Moving

However great the pressure to get to your destination, if you are driving long-distance, stop every two hours by the roadside or at a service station, get out of the vehicle, and let your body move.

Stand with your feet hip-width apart, raise your arms from your sides level with your shoulders, then above your head, interlock your fingers, and turn the palms up. Stretching your arms up, bend your knees and drop your pelvis into a squatting position. If you can, roar or groan, then straighten your legs, unclasp your hands, and lower your arms by your sides. Repeat the exercise twice.

Clapping

If you have stopped out in the open air, especially near trees or water, open your lungs to allow them to absorb fresh Qi while stimulating your blood circulation with this simple movement.

Stand with your feet hip-width apart, hands by your sides, swing your arms back and clap your hands behind you, then swing them forward to shoulder level and clap them in front of you. Repeat four times.

Dealing With Aggression

Traveling can be uncomfortable for passengers, but drivers suffer most from long hours sitting in a confined space restricted by a seat belt. To the discomfort must be added tension from the responsibility of driving safely and having to deal with unpredictable behavior and aggression from other drivers. Stress can result, and road rage is occasionally the outcome. Deep, rhythmic breathing, expelling tension in each exhalation, rubbing the hands, gently pinching the ears, stimulating the kidneys, and rotating the feet are simple techniques to dispel fatigue and stay alert. Do them when stuck in traffic jams. On long journeys plan to stop every two hours to stretch and exercise.

Defusing tension

Moving vehicles are dangerous, so tension is rarely absent when driving. It is essential to stop it building up, so that if an emergency of any kind does

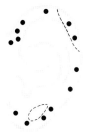

Anmogong ear massage
If you feel tired while traveling, simply pinch all the way around the margins of your ears with your thumbs and index fingers, while breathing deeply and rhythmically through your nose. Pinch fairly gently for up to 30 seconds, then repeat at intervals.

Hand and finger massage
Rub the back of each hand with the palm of the other, then massage each finger. Pay attention to the laogong point at the base of the middle finger, and the soft tissue between the thumb and first finger at the front and back of each hand.

occur, you will be able to deal with it calmly. Being in a car prevents you from stretching your body, but it allows you to stretch the many hundreds of muscles of your face. If there are few other drivers around to see you, or if it is dark, open your mouth wide, stretch it sideways, stick your tongue out. Laugh at yourself. You can make a noise and no one will know: groan, roar, sing loudly. All these activities release tension and defuse aggression.

The program

This program is designed to be performed out of the car during an off-road driving break and will take about ten minutes.

1	Deep breathing (page 210)	1 minute
2	Sitting (page 210)	1 minute
3	Anmogong (page 212):	
	– hands and fingers	30 seconds
	– ears	30 seconds
	– back and kidneys	30 seconds
4	Awaken spine (page 213)	30 seconds
5	Forward bend (page 203)	30 seconds
6	Leg swings (page 62)	30 seconds
7	Clapping (page 211)	30 seconds
8	Knee rotations (page 208)	30 seconds
9	Shaking limbs (page 203)	30 seconds
10	Rainbow circle (pages 190–191)	1 minute

Spinal stretch

If your back aches from prolonged sitting, stop the vehicle, stretch up from the sacrum and place both hands on your back either side of your spine, palms facing your body, one at waist level and the other level with your sacrum. Pressing your palms against your back, rub your hands up and down 20 times. This massages the kidneys, increasing their blood supply and the removal of wastes, and so helps dispel fatigue.

GLOSSARY

crown center or pai hui
The seventh energy center, seated at the top of the head.

taijiquan (t'ai chi ch'uan) A Chinese system of exercises for health and self-development with martial applications; a soft or internal martial art.

dantian (tantien)
Chinese term commonly used to refer to the second energy center, located in the center of the body between the sacrum and a point about 3 inches (7 centimeters) below the navel and also called the lower dantian. The middle dantian, the shanzhong or heart center, is the fourth energy center, and the upper dantian, the yin dantian, also called the brow center or the third eye, is the sixth energy center, located in the middle of the forehead.

Daoism (Taoism) A major Chinese philosophy, thought to have emerged some time before 300 BC, which later evolved into a religion.

dynamic QiGong QiGong exercises that involve making visible movements.

Earthing see **grounding**

form A continuous sequence of choreographed movements.

gateway In QiGong, a part of the body where energy resides or is stored, and through which it can enter or leave the body.

grounding Making and maintaining a strong connection with the center of the Earth and the Earth energy through the legs and feet. Also called Earthing.

heart energy center or shanzhong The fourth energy center, also called the middle dantian, seated in the middle of the chest.

lymph A colorless fluid containing cells called lymphocytes which fight disease. Like the blood, lymph circulates around the body along vessels.

meridians Hidden circuits or channels connecting all parts of the body along which Qi flows.

palm away The palm of the hand is turned away from the body, facing outward.

palm facing The palm of the hand is turned to face inward, toward the body.

perineum The outer layers of muscle and tissue surrounding the urethra and the anus—and the vagina in women—on the floor of the pelvis.

Qi (ch'i or chi) Life force or, literally translated, "life energy." Qi fills the universe and the Earth, and exists in all matter. It circulates around the bodies of living creatures, traveling along channels called meridians.

quiescent QiGong QiGong exercises that involve making no visible movements, such as standing postures and meditations, and so appear static.

QiGong (chi gung or chi kung) A system of exercises for the body and mind that work to build and activate energy or Qi and increase vitality.

root center or hui yin

The first energy center, located at the base of the spine and filling the pelvis. It is called the base or root center because it is the first and lowest of the body's energy gateways.

sacrum A shield-shaped bone made up of five fused bones, which forms the lower spine and the back of the pelvic girdle. The sacrum (literally "sacred bone") forms joints with the fifth lumbar vertebra above, the coccyx or tail bone below, and with the pelvis on either side.

soft To soften the abdomen or any other part of the body is to relax it not only physically but involving the mind in the relaxation process.

solar plexus center or chung wan The third

energy center located in the middle of the body just below the ribs.

step up To make a small adjustment step to move the back foot in toward the front foot.

throat center or shanQi The fifth energy

center located at the front of the neck.

yin and yang General Chinese terms for opposing but complementary forces of nature, representing the female and male principles that govern the universe, alternating in space and time.

FURTHER READING

QIGONG

CHIN, RICHARD M. *The Energy Within*, Paragon House, 1992

DONG, PAUL. *Chi Gong*, Paragon House, 1990

FRANTZIS, BRUCE KUMAR. *Opening the Energy Gates of Your Body*, North Atlantic Books, 1997

KIT, WONG KIEW. *Chi Kung for Health & Vitality*, Element, 1997

REID, DANIEL. *Harnessing the Power of the Universe*, A Comprehensive Guide to the Principles and Practice of QiGong, Simon & Schuster, 1998

REID, DANIEL. *The Tao of Health, Sex and Longevity*, A Fireside Book, New York, 1989

SUN, WEI YUE, AND LI, XIAO JIN. *Chi Kung* Sterling Publishing Co., 1997

WANG, SIMON, AND LIU, JULIUS L. *Qi Gong for Health & Longevity* The East Health Development Group, 1995

CHINESE PHILOSOPHY AND DAOISM

FUNG YU-LAN. *A Short History of Chinese Philosophy*, The Free Press, 1995.

LAO TZU. *Tao Te Ching*, translated by D.C. Lau, Penguin Books, 1998.

LAO TZU. *Tao Te Ching*, translated by Richard Wilhelm, Arkana, 1998.

LAO TZU. *Tao Te Ching*, translated by M.H. Kwok et al, Element Books, 1998.

HEALING

ANODEA, JUDITH. *Wheels of Life*, A User's Guide to the Chakra System, Llewellyn Publications, 1990.

MITCHELL, STEWART. *Naturopathy— Understanding the Healing Power of Nature*, Element Books, 1998.

TAIJIQUAN AND THE MARTIAL ARTS

CHENG MAN-CH'ING. *Cheng Tzu's Thirteen Treatises on Tai Chi Chuan*, translated by Ben Lo and Martin Inn, North Atlantic Books, 1993.

CHENG MAN-CH'ING. *T'ai Chi Ch'uan*, North Atlantic Books, 1993.

CLARK, ANGUS. *The Complete Illustrated Guide to Tai Chi*, Element, 2000

CROMPTON, PAUL. *The Elements of Tai Chi*, Element Books, 1990.

DOCHERTY, DAN. *Complete T'ai Chi Ch'uan*, Crowood Press, 1997.

FINN, MICHAEL. *Martial Arts: A Complete Illustrated History*, Stanley Paul, 1988. Available from Elite Martial Academy, 17A Filmer Road, London SW6 7BU, UK.

LO, BENJAMIN. *The Essence of Tai Chi Chuan: The Literary Tradition*, North Atlantic Books, 1993.

PECK, ALAN. *T'ai Chi: The Essential Introductory Guide*, Vermilion, 1999.

REID, HOWARD, AND CROUCHER, MICHAEL. *The Way of the Warrior* Century Publishing 1983

MAGAZINES

These magazines give useful information about QiGong and taijiquan, list classes, teachers and other contacts, and have interesting articles.

Journal of Asian Martial Arts
Media Publishing Co, 821 West 24th Street, Erie, Pennsylvania 16502
Email: info@goviamedia.com
Web: www.goviamedia.com

Nieuwsbrief published by Stichting Taijiquan Nederland

Qi—The Journal of Traditional Eastern Health and Fitness Insight Graphics Inc, Box 18476, Anaheim Hills, California 92817
Web: www.Qi-journal.com

Qi Magazine PO Box 116, Manchester M20 3YN, UK.
Web: www.Qimagazine.com

Tai Chi—The Leading International Magazine of Tai Chi Chuan Wayfarer Publications, 2601 Silver Ridge Avenue, Los Angeles, California 90039
Web: www.tai-chi.com

Tai Chi and Alternative Health PO Box 6404, London E18 1 EX, UK.Tel: +44 (0)20 8502 9307

T'ai Chi Ch'uan published by the Tai Chi Union for Great Britain

Tai Chi International St Vincent's Publishing, PO Box 460, Thorney, Peterborough, Cambridgeshire PE6 0TQ, UK Tel: +44 (0)1733 270 072
Email: tcinter@easynet.co.uk

Tai Chi Magazine published by the Fédération Française des Tai Chi Chuan Traditionnels

USEFUL ADDRESSES

US

Universal Tai Chi Chuan Association
Contact: Ben Lo
2901 Clement Street,
San Francisco, CA 94121.

William Chen
2 Washington Square Village
#10J, New York, NY 10012.
Tel: +1 (212) 675 2816

The Empty Vessel
Abode of the Eternal Tao
4852 West Amazon
Eugene, OR 97405.
Tel: (800) 574 5118
www.abodetao.com

National QiGong Association *USA
PO Box 540, Ely, MN 55731.
Tel: (218) 365 6933
www.nga.org

QiGong Institute
561Berkeley Avenue
Menlo Park, CA 94025.
www.healthy.net/qigonginstitute

QiGong Association of America
www.qi.org

International Yan Xin QiGong Association
www.qigong.net

Chinese Health Institute
239 Schuyler Avenue
Koingston, PA 18704.
Tel: (570) 287 1316
www.sifuphil.com

Medical QiGong America
PO Box 209
Sandhill, MS 39161.
Tel: (601) 291 4930
www.qigongamerica.com

The QiGong Research Society
199 Sixth Avenue, Mount Laurel
NJ 08054-1010
Tel: (856) 234 3056
www.qigongresearchsociety.com

Toronto Yan Xin QiGong Cultural Centre
188 Main Street
Toronto, Canada
Tel: (416) 699 9216
www.interlog.com/~pparsons/toronto/home.html

Yan Xin QiGong Datong Association
10 Mallory Avenue
Markham, Ontario, Canada
Tel: (905) 477 2621
http://home.eol.ca

Chinese Da Mo QiGong
http://homepages.go.com/~qigong/qigong.htm

HOLISTIC VACATIONS/RETREATS

These three centers regularly offer QiGong in their programs. All are located in Europe but have an international reputation.

Skyros Holistic Vacations
Skyros, Greece
Tel: +44 (0) 171 267 4424
Skyros@easynet.co.uk
www.skyros.com

La Serranía
Mallorca, Spain
Tel: +34 (0) 639 306 432
Fax +34 (0) 971 182 144
www.laserrania.com

Cortijo Romero
Spain
bookings@cortijo-romero.co.uk
www.cortijo-romero.co.uk

Ashburton Centers,
79 East Street,
Ashburton, Devon TQ3 7AL
Tel: +44 (0) 1364 652784
www.ashburtoncenter.co.uk

US

Dreamweaver Lodge
PO Box 1686
Red Lodge, MT 59068
Tel: (406) 445 2517
www.dreamweaverlodge.com

CHINESE TERMS

Chinese is a language with no alphabet and many sounds unknown in English and European languages, and there are many different systems for transliterating it. Until recently, the Wade-Giles system was usually used in British English and the Yale system in American English. These different systems explain the confusing differences in the way Chinese words are spelled in English. For example, under the Wade-Giles system, "QiGong" is written "chi kung" and under the Yale system "chi gung." In 1958 a new system, called pinyin, was officially adopted by the Chinese government. This is now extensively used in education and by the media in China and in the West. In pinyin, "chi kung" or "chi gung" is written "QiGong," "chi" is written "Qi," and "tao" and "Taoism" as "dao" and "Daoism." The official sanctioning of the pinyin system explains why we now write Mao Zedong and Beijing instead of Mao Tse-tung or Mao Tse Tung and Peking. It will be many years, however, before pinyin is universally understood, so in this book we have used the new, official spelling and, where we feel it may be helpful we have inserted the old spelling in parenthesis after the new one: taijiquan (t'ai chi ch'uan). The names of people who became well known before the 1950s are spelled in the old way.

INDEX

ACKNOWLEDGMENTS

Special thanks go to Kay Macmullan, C. A. Stone, and R. Dench
for help with photography.

PICTURE ACKNOWLEDGMENTS

Every effort has been made to trace copyright holders and obtain permission.
The publishers apologize for any omissions and would be pleased
to make any necessary changes at subsequent printings

AKG, London 18B, 35, 128;
The Art Archive, London 14, 38;
Corbis, London / 8 Galen Rowell, 19T Brian Vikander,
27L Tom Nebbia, 38 Earl and Nazima Kowall;
The Image Bank, London 200;
Stone/Getty One 210.

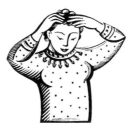